FITNESS WITHOUT EXERCISE

SHAPES UP WELL WITH THE EXPERTS

"Stamford and Shimer have the moxie to tell the truth—that most systematic exercise is damnably boring—and that anything you do as a matter of duty and not fun is probably bad for you. This is not to say that there aren't many people who like to do sitting-up exercises or stationary bicycles or aerobics in front of a TV screen. This book isn't trying to deflect them or discourage them. Rather, it's intended for those people who would rather do things that really interest them. The big news is that these people can stay off their rowing machines or jogging track and still be healthy. For Stamford and Shimer recognize that good health is mostly a matter of lifestyle, of nutrition, of what we do with our minds, how we handle our stresses, how we tend to our hearts, and how we make ourselves useful in the world. In all these respects, Stamford and Shimer have provided things of ultimate value."

—Norman Cousins
bestselling author of *The Healing Heart* and *Head First*

*

"Stamford and Shimer's recommendations for moderate exercise and a low-fat diet are right on target. I'm pleased that they're spreading the good word."

—Martin Katahn
bestselling author of *The Rotation Diet* and *The T-Factor Diet*

*

"*Fitness Without Exercise* contains information on how to become fit for life that will surprise most people and benefit everyone. I wish this book were required reading in high schools across the United States. Young people need to know this information; their lives depend on it! But no matter what your age, this book will guide you in the right direction."

—Bill Rodgers
multiple winner of the New York and Boston marathons

*

"Totally original, glistening with fresh insights . . . I have chosen exercise every day of my adult life, but it is great to know that there are alternative ways to good health that are both fun and effective. Those who chafe at regimented exercise routines will be delighted to find here a get-in-shape strategy that is as good for the soul as it is for the body."

—Wayne Dyer
author of *Your Erroneous Zones*
and *You'll See It When You Believe It*

"This wonderful book represents a milestone in the American self-health movement. First, because it argues convincingly that those of us with exercise-on-the-brain need desperately to readjust our state of mind. And second, because it demonstrates that maximum wellness is easily achieved when living and exercising run confluently one into the other. I intend to prescribe this book to all of my patients."

—Gideon Bosker, M.D.
editorial board, *American Journal of Medicine*

*

"Refreshingly pointed and on the mark. . . . It's conversant, non-technical, scientifically based and utterly useful to all those individuals out there who have for years been duped into a lifestyle of pain, boredom and senseless—mindless—running, stretching and pumping iron in the name of health and fitness. . . . The point is clear. Training can be fun—it is for me—but . . . if it isn't for you, then do yourself a real service and read what Stamford and Shimer have to say. They have a lot to say, and they say it ever so well."

—Frederick C. Hatfield, Ph.D.
former powerlifting world record holder and current
senior VP and director, Research and Development,
Weider Health & Fitness, Inc.

*

"With wit and good, clean prose Stamford and Shimer point out what should be self-evident but isn't to many American treadmillers: fitness can and should be fun, not a job, and as personalized and integral to our lives as the clothes we put on in the morning. Every body-perfect proselytizer in the land should be forced to sit stone-still in a chair and read this book through a week of workouts."

—Charles Gaines
bestselling author of *Pumping Iron*

*

"*Fitness Without Exercise* is a timely warning. . . . It challenges the idea that we can measure good health through athletic performance, pointing out that people who tend their gardens may benefit as much as 10K runners."

—Rona Cherry
editor-in-chief, *Longevity* magazine

*

"*Fitness Without Exercise* candidly slashes through the overplayed and unsubstantiated fitness myths, too often ill-founded on duty and guilt, and releases the neglected truths of a totally healthy lifestyle. I am convinced that Stamford and Shimer's powerful message, which emphasizes striking a balance among mental attitude, nutritional observance, and moderate activity, is the only answer to counter the ravages of heart, lung, and vessel disease which I battle daily as a heart and lung surgeon. *Fitness Without Exercise* contains the right prescription for the nineties."

—William H. Frist, M.D.   director, Heart-Lung Transplantation,
Vanderbilt University Medical Center, and author of *Transplant*

FITNESS WITHOUT EXERCISE

The scientifically proven strategy for achieving maximum health with minimum effort

BRYANT A. STAMFORD, PH.D.
PORTER SHIMER

WARNER BOOKS

A Warner Communications Company

Copyright © 1990 by Bryant A. Stamford, Ph.D., and Porter Shimer

Warner Books, Inc., 666 Fifth Avenue, New York, NY 10103

w A Warner Communications Company

Printed in the United States of America

First printing: March 1990

10 9 8 7 6 5 4 3 2 1

Library of Congress Cataloging-in-Publication Data
Stamford, Bryant A.
    Fitness without exercise / Bryant A. Stamford, Porter Shimer.
        p.   cm.
    Includes bibliographical references.
    ISBN 0-446-51537-X
    1. Health.   2. Physical fitness.   3. Exercise.   4. Low-fat diet.
I. Shimer, Porter.   II. Title.
RA776.5.S73   1990
613—dc20   89-40457
                                                              CIP

Book design by H. Roberts

To Joy Donaldson-Stamford, my wife and my best friend, and to my sons, Bryant and Benjamin

—Bryant A. Stamford

To all fitness avoiders, fitness addicts, and fitness flops, may you find your way. And to Richard Pine and Rick Horgan, the Lone Ranger and Tonto of publishing, thanks for the justice

—Porter Shimer

ACKNOWLEDGMENTS

I am indebted to Joy Donaldson-Stamford, my wife, for her many contributions to this book. Some contributions are easily recognized—the recipe section, for example. Others are hidden. She offered fresh perspectives on stale issues. She boosted my morale when needed, and her constructive criticism was always crisp and meaningful.

I am deeply grateful to the many people I've come to know in the past few years who are labeled mentally retarded. They have shown me the wisdom of living in the moment and accepting with grace what life has to offer. This book would not have been conceived without their contributions to my thinking.

I thank Linda Ward, my administrative assistant, for her encouragement and delightful sense of humor. She is a great asset to my work and a good friend. And I am indebted to Georgia Alice Stamford, my mother, for sleuthing a wide variety of lay press publications in an effort to keep me up to date—especially on topics of interest to gerontologists. She is forever dependable.

I acknowledge the help of Richard Pine, our agent. His support and optimism provided a much-needed boost to our confidence.

Finally, I acknowledge the contributions of Rick Horgan, senior editor at Warner Books. He believed in our ideas from the outset, and he worked very hard to bring this book into being.

—Bryant A. Stamford

Thanks to my family (Connie, Elizabeth, Sarah, Mom and Pop, Bob, Andy, Gretchen, Sonia, Judy and Ed) and all my friends at Rodale Press.

—Porter Shimer

CONTENTS

Part III: Nutrition and Weight Control: Eat Better, Weigh Less

Part IV: Closing Remarks: Push-ups for the Personality

REQUIEM FOR THE SWEAT SUIT

It came trying to help us,
And for some it succeeded.
But for more than it helped,
It chafed and defeated.

Can fitness be gained without such a suit?
Can long life be reached by a more pleasing route?

Take heart, yes it can.
Sweat is not gold.
Purpose and joy
Give the strength to grow old.

—Porter Shimer

PROLOGUE: For Whom This Book Tolls

This book tolls for Mary Ann, who's more concerned about raising her three children than her maximal oxygen uptake.

It tolls for George, who'd rather work on his 1939 Ford than his "biceps."

It tolls for Ted, whose dedication to the triathlon has cost him a marriage and a job.

This book, in short, tolls for all whom the fitness movement has missed but also for those it has kidnapped.

Introduction: A Challenge to Colleagues

When we decided to write this book, we knew full well the reaction its title would get from you, our colleagues in the fields of exercise physiology and health promotion.

"New heights in fitness quackery. These guys should be roped to a treadmill until they repent or until they drop."

To which we say, "We'll run your treadmill if you'll just read our book." We're confident that if you do, you'll come away with a fresh perspective that will change the way you look at your work.

What we propose in the pages ahead makes more sense than the fitness movement has been able to make in twenty years. The latest figures show that only 10 to 15 percent of American adults engage regularly in enough aerobic exercise to qualify as "fit" according to current American College of Sports Medicine standards. Some surveys indicate our fitness levels may even be declining, since participation in such "hard-core" conditioning activities as jogging, swimming, racquetball, and aerobics has fallen off since 1984. Surveys also show that we're getting fatter. The average American adult has put on about 6 pounds of fat since 1980.

We'll be presenting more grim details on the failure of the fitness movement in our first chapter, but the point we wish to make here is simply that it may be time for a different approach to the fitness problem. If twenty years haven't worked, why should twenty more, especially if most recent surveys show us to be heading in the wrong direction? As health professionals, we all need to rethink what it is we've really been trying to accomplish with our exercise emphasis. Has it been to endorse exercise simply for the sake of exercise?

Of course not. What we've been trying to do in advocating exercise is to arrest specific health problems—i.e., the heart attacks, hypertension, diabetes, strokes, and obesity that have ravaged this country since the beginning of the Industrial Revolution. If we could find a way to do that without aerobic exercise, we'd abandon our aerobic ideals in a minute, would we not?

Well, get ready to jump ship, because there is such a way. Yes, a

1

regular aerobic exercise program can help defend against all the lifestyle-related diseases mentioned above, but so can a prudent low-fat diet, *modest* physical activity, and learning to keep the lid on bad habits and stress. To the degree that adherence to a regular aerobic exercise program has allowed some people to think they can slight these other health factors, in fact, the exercise movement has done as much damage, perhaps, as good. The marathon runner, for example, who feels he earns exemption from a diet high in fat is running dangerously from the truth. Deceived, too, is the high-powered executive who believes that the cardiovascular hazards imposed by a hostile, mad dash for success can be erased by playing racquetball three times a week. We need to let these people know their folly before it's too late.

And to do that we need a new concept of fitness, one that is less physically and athletically demanding. In the book that's been credited with giving the fitness kick its start—*Aerobics*—Ken Cooper determined that fitness is the ability to run a mile and a half in no more than twelve minutes. What does that say for the vegetarian with flat feet who has a cholesterol level of only 120, a blood pressure of 100/70, less than 15 percent body fat, and a great attitude about life—that he needs to join a health club?

We propose a new concept of fitness, one that is more lenient physically than Cooper's, but one that is more encompassing, more healthful, and more strict in other ways. We propose, for example, that the amount of fat in the diet and that such vital statistics as cholesterol levels, blood pressure, and percentage of body fat be deemed more important than one's aerobic power, and we propose that mental outlook be an important consideration as well. Anyone who's got all those cards in order doesn't have to worry about a mile and a half run.

The fitness movement has done little to improve the health of the masses and the reason is simple: Emphasis has been placed on improving physical performance, and improved physical performance is not something most Americans want or need.

It's time we shifted the fitness emphasis away from performance and more toward health and well-being, and if you think there's little or no distinction here, you're one of the reasons we wrote this book. The difference is great, and its significance must not be underestimated if we are going to reverse the tide of lifestyle diseases that plague us.

Please don't misunderstand us, however. We don't come here to bury exercise, only to redefine it so that its benefits are made more accessible to those who need it most. We'll show that physical activity short of producing a "target heart rate" can substantially reduce the risk of heart disease, just as we'll show that a "fit" attitude about life and a "fit" diet can do the same. Expect to see *special emphasis* on diet, in fact, because we feel very strongly that it has been the missing link in the fitness movement's assault on heart attacks so far. We've coined a new phrase, in fact—"lipo-fitness"—which we feel encompasses an important point that the aerobics movement has missed. Virtually all of the major "diseases of lifestyle" that the exercise movement has tried to combat can *just as effectively* be deterred by a low-fat, high-fiber diet rich in complex carbohydrates. The fitness movement has badly missed the point in this regard. The best way to keep fat out of the arteries is to keep it out of the mouth, and a low-fat diet also can greatly reduce risks of high blood pressure, diabetes, obesity, and blood-clotting that can lead to strokes. We'll be looking at all of these features of lipo-fitness later in this book.

But lipo-fitness aside, what about the *psychological* benefits of aerobic exercise—the feelings of accomplishment and confidence and the relief from stress that can come from a good sweat? How are dietary changes going to substitute for those?

For the rare few who really get those kinds of rewards from a hard workout, we say, "Great." Keep it up, because less fat in the diet is *not* going to provide those gifts. The truth, however, is that most people are intimidated and humbled by the rigors of an aerobic workout, so for them we offer a different kind of exercise experience entirely, one that can strengthen the heart and burn calories, but not at the expense of motivation. Just as much pride and stress relief can come from tending a garden as from reducing one's time in a 10-kilometer race. Just as much of a "high" can be had from remodeling one's family room as from remodeling one's abdominals.

Beginning to get the picture? It's time we stopped trying to train John and Mary Doe as though the rat race were a track meet. Emotional fitness and dietary fitness are every bit as important, if not more important, than performance fitness, and this country's 200 million "fitness failures" deserve to know.

See you at the treadmill.

—Bryant A. Stamford, Ph.D.

Porter Shimer

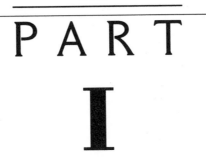

PART
I

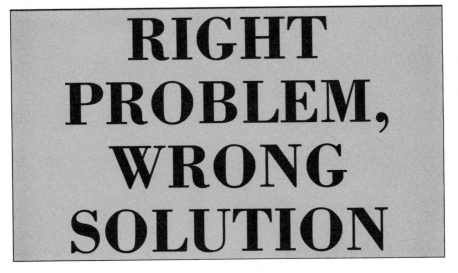

RIGHT PROBLEM, WRONG SOLUTION

—

1

Why the Fitness Boom Has Been a Bust

Shimer

Beware of all enterprises that require new clothes.
—Henry David Thoreau, 1817–1862

When Dr. Ken Cooper introduced his concept of "aerobic" exercise more than twenty years ago, America suddenly had itself what seemed like a perfect drug. Not only could the drug combat heart disease, high blood pressure, diabetes, obesity, osteoporosis, and stress, but it could also produce a mild "high." Even the drug's one drawback, a fairly stiff requirement of effort, worked in its favor at first because the effort relieved guilt. You could feel better about the hot dogs, the apple pie, and new Chevrolet if you paid your aerobic "dues."

And indeed, some dues were due. The Kennedy administration had just finished berating us for letting the fitness levels of our school children fall to new lows, and all we had to do was look in the mirror to see where they were getting their inspiration. Add the reprimands that were coming from the medical community regarding new records being set for virtually all obesity-related disorders (fatal heart attacks, high blood pressure, diabetes, and strokes), and it's easy to see why we reached for Dr. Cooper's aerobic medicine with such gusto.

But has the medicine worked?

Unfortunately, it has not. Despite what the athletic shoe and yogurt commercials would have us believe, only 10 to 15 percent of U.S. adults currently do enough exercise (at least three twenty-minute workouts a week that sustain a target heart rate of at least 60 percent of maximum) to qualify as aerobically "fit" according to standards set by the American College of Sports Medicine (ACSM). The rest of us either have attempted a fitness program and failed, or we have chosen simply to ignore the fitness call entirely.

Yes, fatal heart attacks seem finally to be on the decline. but the drop is being credited less to aerobic exercise than to other factors—improved screening and treatment of heart disease, better drugs for controlling high blood pressure and serum cholesterol, and less smoking. The fitness movement has failed even in its fight against obesity as an all-time high of four out of ten adults currently carry around at least 20 percent more of themselves than they should. Even the commercial strength of the fitness movement is withering. Sales of exercise equipment have been on a downward spiral since 1985, and record numbers of health clubs are being forced to throw in the towel daily.

Where did the movement go wrong? How could such energetic personalities as Charles Atlas, Jack LaLanne, Jim Fixx, Jackie Sorensen, Jane Fonda, and Richard Simmons come but not conquer?

There are a variety of answers to that question. Aerobic exercise has been accused of being too boring, too time-consuming, and too strenuous. It's our belief, however, that two other factors have been more responsible for the movement's breakdown. The crusade has failed, first of all, by not allowing exercise to be practical. Jogging does not help pay the mortgage or clean the rain gutters, just as riding a stationary bicycle does not get the wash done or help make dinner for the kids. Not a single exercise currently endorsed by the fitness establishment is capable of producing anything other than sweat. For a nation raised on the practical wisdoms of Ben Franklin and the work ethics of Horatio Alger, that's been hard to accept. We're a society that likes to be rewarded for its labors, and concerned though we may be about our health and the way we look, those concerns pale next to our needs for financial security and material comfort as measured by the almighty dollar.

But the fitness movement has failed for being more than just impractical; it's failed for being no fun. Yes, the aerobic dance people came along and said, "Crank up the stereo," but they also said, "Crank up the heart rate, and be sure to steal at least thirty to forty-five minutes three times a week to do it." The party quickly lost favor.

Research on exercise adherence shows that the majority of people who embark on a three-workout-a-week aerobic program don't last more than a few months, and only a small fraction last more than a year. We're a society whose sense of time urgency is very great and whose intolerance for boredom is even greater. The combination has made the idea of sitting on a stationary bicycle or rowing machine for ninety minutes a week seem less like a health effort than a punishment.

Perhaps even more disturbing, however, has been the fitness movement's lack of impact on our children. Efforts of the Kennedy administration notwithstanding, the majority of American children between the ages of six and seventeen qualify as "unfit" according to minimal standards of cardiovascular endurance and muscular strength. Worse yet, 40 percent of children between the ages of five and eight demonstrate at least one major risk factor for heart disease—elevated serum cholesterol, high blood pressure, or obesity. Our kids are accumulating strikes against them before even stepping up to the plate.

A Call for Lower Standards

The failure of the fitness movement has been severe enough for Kenneth E. Powell, M.D., of the Centers for Disease Control in Atlanta, to suggest that we try a whole new approach to the fitness problem. Dr. Powell recently called for a re-examination of the goals set forth by the Public Health Service in 1980—goals that anticipated 60 percent of American adults engaging in three aerobic workouts a week by the year 1990. We're so far from that objective at this point that Dr. Powell is suggesting we lower our standards. "We've considered each 1990 objective and what's been learned since those objectives were made," he recently announced. "We're suggesting that maybe they're too high, that maybe there are good benefits [to be had] at lower levels of activity."

Don't get us wrong—the fitness movement has meant well and for many it has done great things. Millions of people have used regular exercise to improve their appearance, boost their self-confidence, and improve their health. Where the movement has done so many of us a disservice, however, has been in painting a needlessly stark picture of how this thing called "fitness" must be earned—through miles jogged, laps swum, sit-ups sat. Especially hard to accommodate has been the concept of the "target heart rate"—getting the heart beating to within 60 to 90 percent of its maximum and *keeping it there* for a minimum of twenty to thirty minutes at least three times and preferably four or five times a week.

Has this formula been cited to suggest that anything less goes for naught? That someone who expends 500 calories on a Saturday afternoon reshingling his roof gets no cardiovascular credit because his heart rate averages 50 percent instead of 60, or because he stops too often to wave to his kids or enjoy the view? Has the formula been used to imply that calories burned running a vacuum cleaner or washing windows somehow count less than those burned by doing jumping jacks at a health club?

Yes, that's exactly what the "fitness" formula has implied and it's why fitness has flopped. We've been given the impression that if we can't get exercise in the right amounts or at the right intensities, we might as well not get any at all. It's been that kind of thinking that has driven millions of us to upgrade our TVs and go down for the count. Others have put up a little more of a struggle, but with essentially the same results. We figured we'd weed out the meaningless exercise from our lives to gain more time for the "real" thing. Walt, for example, traded his 22-inch push-type lawnmower for a 48-inch ride-on model with hopes of taking up jogging. He should have checked first with his knees. Or Janet—she hired a house cleaner so she could join a health club. She now has guilt to pay in addition to the membership and the maid. Our fitness quest at its worst has made Don Quixote look competent. We'll park in a "reserved for the handicapped" zone at the supermarket because we're in a hurry to get home to do leg lifts with our latest exercise video, then watch a "M*A*S*H" rerun instead. We'll ride escalators in search of the right color athletic shoes.

Is there a way out of this fitness farce? Is there a way we can have our careers, our families, our hobbies, our well-kept homes and yet our weight control, healthy hearts, and *la joie de vivre*, too?

Yes, and that's what this book is about. Our dilemma appears complex, but its solution is actually quite simple. For starters, we've got to learn to appreciate the value of physical activity that has nothing to do with putting on a sweat suit or counting sit-ups, push-ups, or heart rates. We've got to realize that there's health to be had in simple around-the-house chores and in simple pleasures such as a game of badminton or a leisurely stroll to watch the sunset. New research is showing that not only have the austere standards of the aerobics crusade been tough to meet, but they've been downright wrong. Simple movement can help protect against heart disease whether it produces a "target heart rate" or not. Exercise gotten in bits and pieces can "count" as much as exercise gotten in large sweat-producing chunks. Body fat can be burned by walking a dog as well as by running a marathon.

Where's the proof?

In some very convincing pudding. Several epidemiological (population-based) studies have come out recently—and we suspect more will be reaching print before this book does—showing that physical activity does not have to be vigorous or extensive to achieve sizable health gains. As Dr. Steven N. Blair, of the Institute for Aerobics Research in Dallas, has remarked regarding these new studies, which we'll be looking at in more detail shortly, "It doesn't take an enormous amount of activity to obtain considerable health benefits." The message seems to be "get up, turn off the TV, move around, do some gardening, or go for a walk."

The new wave of fitness research has scientists looking at even some of the older studies in a new light—the 1978 study of 17,000 Harvard alumni by Dr. Ralph Paffenbarger, for example, which has been credited with giving the fitness movement a big boost. The study found that exercise levels of 2,000 calories a week afforded significant protection from heart disease, but what early interpretations of the data failed to point out was how most of those 2,000 calories were being burned. It was not through aerobic activities such as jogging, but rather from simple day-to-day activities such as walking, stair climbing, and light sports.

Another misleading interpretation of the Paffenbarger data was that significant health benefits did not begin to accrue until the minimal 2,000 calories worth of exercise a week had been reached. But this, too, has been shown to be wrong. As Dr. Ronald LaPorte, of the University of Pittsburgh, has since interpreted the data, "If you draw a graph of the health benefits versus sweat invested, you see increasing health benefits as activity rises from 500 calories a week (which is just about comatose) to 3,500 calories. The line rises sharply on this graph from 500 to 2,000 calories, but from 2,000 to 3,500—the fitness range—the returns flatten out. Everybody's been concentrating on the high end of the graph, but the greatest health returns actually show up at the 'low' end."

Be aware, however, that although 500 calories a week of physical activity can provide modest health benefits, it's not enough to help avoid heart attack. Dr. William Haskell, of Stanford University, concluded from his review of relevant literature that a minimal threshold of 1,050 calories per week of physical activity is required to decrease heart disease risk— that's 150 calories a day. So the range you need to shoot for is from the minimum of 1,050 calories per week to the optimum of 2,000 calories per week.

Gain Without Pain

The new research offers encouraging news, because it indicates there's a lot more room on the fitness bandwagon than anyone previously thought. There's room for Jake, who'd rather swing a hammer than swim laps, and there's room for his wife, Karen, who'd rather grow vegetables than jog. There's room for Walt, whose ride-on lawn mower was leaving tire marks in his yard, anyway, and there's room for Janet, whose housecleaner was doing her best work on the cookie jar. There's even room for all you well-heeled professionals who've been avoiding lunchtime walks thinking they have to leave you drenched in a sweat to do any good.

Miles jogged and toes touched?

Why not leaves raked and laundry hung to dry? Elevators avoided and taxis not taken? We have a chance for a whole new way of playing the fitness ballgame, and it's especially good news for anyone not opposed to saving a nickel. Greater self-sufficiency can help us burn calories instead of cash.

Gain can be had without pain, in other words, and you don't only get what you sweat for. That might sound like health heresy to the fitness missionaries who've been pushing perspiration at us for more than twenty years, but the new, softer dogma has plenty of science on its side. Yes, there are benefits to regular aerobic "workouts," but the benefits do not appear to be significantly greater than those to be gained by simple "work"—or by simple "play," for that matter. What's even more significant is that the benefits of aerobic exercise appear to be minor compared to what scientists are now learning about the effects of diet, stress control, the positive effects of happiness, and the negative effects of anger, hostility, and the ubiquitous vices of tobacco, alcohol, and drugs.

The image of the marathon runner living to be ninety despite a diet of junk food and beer, however, dies hard. We've been led to believe that exercise turns the digestive system into a blast furnace capable of decimating any dietary disaster man can concoct, but it's just not so. A high-fat diet can claim the heart of the marathoner, whether he qualifies for Boston or not. We've got to realize that perhaps the most direct route of all to better health is not via the muscles, but via the mouth.

Nor is exercise necessarily a guard against stress; for some it's even a contributor. The fact that "no pain, no gain" has survived as the fitness movement's rallying cry as long as it has would suggest that the movement's policy makers have been woefully slow to understand the very real hazards of the "more is better" lifestyle. It seems unfortunate to us that the average American should see nothing incongruous about rushing home from work to get to an unenjoyably exhausting exercise class and then feel justified in taking a reward of a double-bacon cheeseburger.

But such has been the fitness fiasco. Exercise has been portrayed as the universal elixir, the magic bullet. Bite it hard for best results. The more it hurts, the more it heals. After twenty years, however, the naïveté of that thinking has finally been exposed. There are all too many superbly conditioned athletes with serious alcohol and drug problems. Many regular exercisers remain addicted to cigarettes. And many people who are lonely or hostile seek refuge in the simple, safe, and predictable world of exercise. But a sanctuary it is not. At best it's a temporary shelter from the storm, an analgesic whose pain-killing effects are short-lived. And at worst it's a powerful narcotic capable of distorting priorities and becoming master rather than servant.

"Go for the burn or don't bother"?

If you're ready for an end to that sort of health club hogwash, come on along. We'll show you an easier, more enjoyable, more natural, more practical, *and more effective* way.

2

The Reformation of an Exercise Addict

Stamford

For the unquiet heart and brain. . . .
the sad mechanic exercise,
like dull narcotics, numbing pain.
—Alfred Tennyson, 1809–1892

The sweat gear is still damp from the day before. A voice on the radio announces a wind chill factor of −10 degrees F. It's 5:35 A.M. But I suit up anyway, afraid I won't have time later.

Do I want to?

Of course not.

Do I feel I have to for health reasons?

No.

Do I see anything to be gained from this run at all?

Yes, I do. I see freedom from the guilt of not doing it.

It was that realization that forced me to make the first U-turn of my life that fateful morning in December. About a mile out, I hit a patch of ice and went down, hard. Normally I'd have bounced up quickly, my only worry being whether I had let my heart rate slow down. But this time I felt paralyzed. I wasn't injured physically, but my spirit felt destroyed. For the first time in more than twenty years of daily workouts, I knew I would not be able to get up and conquer the sense of utter absurdity in what I was doing.

I felt defeated, beaten by my own impossible standards. I had done it to myself, of course, but that didn't make the sense of defeat any less devastating. How would I conduct myself as the Director of the Exercise

13

Physiology Laboratory at the University of Louisville that day? How would I feel as I sat down to write my weekly health and fitness column for the *Louisville Courier-Journal* that night? How would I ever be able to face the participants in my adult fitness class in the spring?

As I slowly made my way back home that morning, I was tempted several times to resume my run and write the whole experience off as a close call. But I knew it had been much more than that. It had been the culmination of doubts I'd been having for years. Exercise was supposed to be an antidote for stress—I preached that in my writings and taught it in my classes—but for me it had become an immense source of stress, a bully that I knew would be beating me up daily. Exercise also was supposed to be an energizer—I preached that, too—but for me it had become a monumental drain. My workouts left me feeling numb. Sometimes I would experience a slight uplift in mood after a workout, but only because the whipping was over. It was only a matter of time before I'd begin to feel anxious and depressed as the next flogging grew near.

I was a prisoner of fitness, a man shackled by his own dedication to a cause that had lost its purpose. I had pain in several joints in my body from old sports and fitness injuries. I lacked the energy and motivation to do simple chores around the house. I felt forever short of time because of the hours my addiction was stealing. And I called myself fit?

I was a cripple. But at least I was a cripple who knew what he had to do. I had to quit exercising—cold turkey. I knew I wouldn't be able just to cut back—my addiction was too severe. I had to dry out completely before I could even think about imbibing again. I needed a clean and sober perspective that only total abstinence could give.

Was it tough?

It was murder, a lot more grueling than any workout. I experienced anxiety, depression, self-doubt, and guilt. I was irritable and short-tempered. I would pass joggers on the road and feel resentful that they could enjoy what I could not.

But gradually things changed. Several weeks into my rehabilitation, I began experiencing a sense of liberation I had never known as an adult. I now had options. Every minute was not accounted for on a rigid timetable dictated by exercise. My days no longer seemed too short. I was getting to work and keeping appointments on time—with ease. I could eat a meal without worrying whether it would have time to digest before my next workout. I could wake up in the morning without fear and dread. I could go to sleep at night without feeling like a victim. I had energy. I felt free!

But was I cured? After several months I began wondering if I could return to exercise without once again becoming its slave. I knew physical activity had benefits—it had been my fault for taking it to damaging extremes. Was I now strong enough to drink without getting drunk?

I had to find out. I started with short walks, making sure not to chart distance or time. I made it a point to climb stairs, making sure not to count how many or how often. I even spent time in a weight room—and left without fretting about how much I had lifted and for how many reps. The number monkey was off my back!

I began to look at household chores in a whole new light. In the old days I resisted jobs around the house because they weren't strenuous enough to qualify as "exercise." I would do them, if at all, only after I had worked out, and then half-heartedly. But now I'd developed a new attitude toward work as "exercise that makes sense." I'd become a veritable white tornado—something between Mr. Universe and Mr. Clean—and my wife and neighbors much preferred me for it.

How did this new attitude toward fitness affect my physique? That had been a major concern of mine going into this "rehab" period, I must confess, but it also turned out to be a major surprise. Despite changing from an exercise fanatic to little better than a handyman virtually overnight, my body barely seemed to notice. I'm not going to say my peak aerobic capacity remained as high as it had been, but my weight did not change, my appearance did not change, my blood pressure did not change, and my serum cholesterol actually dropped, the result of my new approach to diet. (As an exercise abuser, I used to think I could get away with being a human garbage disposal.)

Perhaps the greatest and most welcome benefit to come from my exercise "liberation," however, has been the boost in energy—mental as well as physical. It's clear to me now that I'd simply been drawing too much from the bucket. If physical fitness had been my livelihood, as it is for some Olympic and professional athletes, the fatigue could have been justified. But I was trying to be a husband, a father, a teacher, a scientist, and superbly fit at the same time, and it just wasn't working.

My new approach to fitness has me feeling more vibrant—mentally as well as physically—than I've ever felt in my life. My weekend hikes leave me ready for something more. My weekend runs, by comparison, used to leave me on the couch, ready for Jim McKay or "NFL Today," at best.

I have found, too, a better type of exercise "high." It's not a runner's high, but a "worker's" high—a deep feeling of satisfaction that comes from having accomplished something other than the mere burning of calories. And for the first time I've allowed myself the luxury of "being" high—the sense of peace and connection that comes from simply walking in a park or down a quiet tree-lined street, experiencing the beauty of nature.

It's occurred to me in the months since my exercise liberation, in fact, that exercise purely for the sake of exercise might be viewed as a waste not just of time, but of food. Sorry, but there seems something regrettably gluttonous to me about an overweight American driving to a health club for the purpose of burning off calories from a meal that might have kept several others in the world alive.

But perhaps the most important consequence of my new independence from structured exercise has come in the context of my professional life. I resigned as Director of the Exercise Physiology Laboratory at the University of Louisville and started a new program called the Health Promotion Center to put my new attitudes about fitness to the test. I also divorced myself from the adult fitness classes I had been teaching and initiated something entirely new: the Health Appraisal—Health Action (HA-HA) that also would reflect my new, less rigorous approach to fitness.

Fitness, I now realized, was not a purely physical phenomenon measurable by one's ability to run on a treadmill. It was a matter of psychological durability and the ability to handle everyday stress. Being physically fit enough to be effective and enthusiastic about running the treadmill called "life" was my new emphasis. The old logic of "no pain, no gain" disappeared down the locker room latrine.

I played down the importance of strenuous aerobic exercise and put enjoyable or purposeful activities in its place. I encouraged people to seek out the variety of opportunities for exercise that surrounded them in their homes, yards, occupational settings, and neighborhood parks. My philosophy was that exercise didn't have to happen in a sweat suit or produce a "target heart rate" to be of value. Any activity was better than no activity, and a premium was placed on practicality and fun.

How did the new approach work out?

Even better than I could have expected. Without emphasis on aerobic exercise, but with increased emphasis on eating better and enjoying life more, people lowered their serum cholesterol levels, they lowered their triglycerides, and they lost body fat. In one class, there was a 12 percent reduction in cholesterol plus other results at least as good as I had been getting in classes with lots of structured exercise. Moreover, class attendance was excellent, much better than in the past, when strenuous exercise was king. Was I onto something?

My work with the Kentucky State Police soon helped answer that. I was hired to assess the fitness/fatness status of troopers and provide guidelines for change. When the project began in 1986, a survey revealed that very few of the approximately 1,000 officers participated in regular exercise of the type and intensity required to produce aerobic fitness. Accordingly, I envisioned a bumper crop of couch potatoes. To my surprise, however, many of the troopers proved to be admirably lean, with good endurance, and they demonstrated low cholesterol and low blood pressure levels as well. Where were they getting their fitness?

Some were getting it spending off-hours tending small farms, I learned. Some were avid firewood cutters. Others were spending a lot of time on "pot patrol"—tramping over hill and dale in search of marijuana plants. They were not, however, doing standardly accepted aerobic exercise, and yet they had respectable fitness/fatness and health profiles.

I barely had time to contemplate the implications of my findings when the news hit: A report in the November 6, 1987, *Journal of the American Medical Association* confirming the importance of the discovery I had made personally as well as in working with others. A multiyear study coordinated by Arthur Leon, M.D., and colleagues from the University of Minnesota School of Public Health had found that "men at high risk for CHD (coronary heart disease) who self-selected moderate amounts of predominately light and moderate nonwork physical activity had lower rates of CHD mortality, sudden death, and overall mortality than more sedentary men." A modest amount of physical activity is a whole lot better than none at all, in other words. But the major finding of the study was that men who engaged in at least thirty minutes daily of "moderate leisure time physical activity" were enjoying the same protection from fatal heart attacks as men whose exercise levels were three times that much.

A major victory for walkers, gardeners, golfers, homekeepers, and "Mr. Fixits" had been won. Activities considerably below the aerobic threshold for raising heart rate and taxing the cardiovascular system had been found not to be "wastes of time" after all. Had a step beyond aerobics been found?

These were precisely my thoughts when I got a phone call from Porter Shimer, the editor of a health and fitness newsletter for which I'm an advisor.

"There's something happening here," Porter said of the newly published report.

"I know," I said, "I've found the same results in my own work. But how do you communicate a message like this to a society that's still in a craze about fitness?"

"I think the craze is on the verge of a crash," Porter answered. "People have been made to feel inadequate by the rigors of the aerobic system long enough. They're ready for a better way."

I agreed and this book was born.

The Case of the Dangling Heart

As I began to pull together thoughts and data that spanned more than twenty years, I was struck by the magnitude of the change in my thinking. I had been a zealot, a defender of the faith—the jogger's jogger who fought proudly in defense of a cherished belief. The following "confrontation" illustrates my point.

In 1975, an article entitled "Jogging May Be Hazardous to Your Health" appeared in the Saturday magazine section of the Louisville newspaper. The essay by J. E. Schmidt, M.D., began as follows: "Running or jogging may be one of the most wasteful and hazardous forms of exercise for both men and women. Jogging takes more from the body than it gives . . . it exacts a price that no one can afford or should be willing to pay. . . ."

Step by step, Dr. Schmidt chronicled gruesome atrocities. Jogging ravages the body from all points—north, south, east, and west, he argued. Starting at the base of the spine, where the effects of jogging on the pelvis are "not unlike the splitting of a log by driving a wedge into its crevice with a sledge hammer," jogging moves next to the vertebrae of the spine, where it "contributes to the condition of a slipped disk . . . by providing the disk with an hydraulic impact at each step. . . ."

Jogging is not content just with skeletal damage, however. It jars sludge out of the veins and causes clots and crusts to be swept into the heart and lungs, Schmidt said. And because the heart is not well anchored inside the chest cavity, Schmidt claimed that jogging treats that vital organ much as an automobile accident would, where "the body is suddenly stopped by a collision" and "the heart breaks through the chest wall and remains suspended grotesquely outside by its blood vessels, like an old light fixture detached from the ceiling and hanging awkwardly on its wires."

As if that weren't enough to take the fun out of a fun run, Schmidt added the danger of hernia pushing through the abdominal wall "like a ladleful of cooked spaghetti in a greased funnel."

"Nor are these the only casualties of jogging," he concluded. "Among the others are dropped stomach, loose spleen, floating kidney, and fallen arches." Women, especially, needed to keep off the jogging paths, Schmidt said, lest they be willing to see their uterus dislodged and their breasts "droop like a partly deflated balloon."

As both an exercise physiologist at the University of Louisville and a fitness instructor, I was aghast, to say the least. I wrote a rebuttal to the newspaper, which was printed two weeks later, but it didn't attract a fraction of the attention captured by Dr. Schmidt's expose. To thousands of readers, Schmidt had come off as a savior, a much welcomed voice of authority saying, "Roll that Lazy Boy back one notch more." I, of course, had been telling people to learn to love the smell of sweat.

Eventually Schmidt and I wound up going head to head on a local TV news show, and the meeting was as spirited as might be expected. I tried to make the point that if the internal organs were indeed as poorly suspended as Dr. Schmidt claimed, then surely the innards of football players, springboard divers, parachute jumpers, and trampoline artists must look like stewed tomatoes. Things got hot and the moderator loved it.

But a lot can happen in fourteen years. I look back now with respect for what Dr. Schmidt was trying to do, certainly not out of reverence for his understanding of biology, but rather for his courage to stand up against a movement that was guilty of some gross inaccuracies of its own. Was Dr. Schmidt's image of the dangling heart really any more of an exaggeration than Dr. Thomas Bassler's claim that anyone who can run a marathon is immune to heart disease? The tragic death of Jim Fixx answered that question all too well.

3

The Aerobic Fitness Fallacy

Shimer

Enough is as good as a feast.
—Thomas Heywood, 1497–1580

It's shortly before noon on a Saturday in the backyard of the Petersens' small brick home in Coopersburg, Pennsylvania, and as usual, Father Time is getting no respect at all. Sam, eighty-nine, is cultivating a bumper crop of cabbage while wife, Liz, ninety-one, is tying up some sagging tomato plants. I know because I'm next door riding a stationary bike on my back porch trying to tie up some sagging parts of my own. My name is Porter Shimer, and I've been writing and editing health and fitness newsletters for the Rodale Press since 1978.

I lived next door to the Petersens for eight years, and not once did they fail to have a garden of remarkable bounty. They also succeeded in keeping their lawn as closely cropped as a GI's sideburns. My lawn was lucky to see me three times all year.

The Petersens grew enough vegetables not just for their own needs, but enough to send a lot our way, tomatoes especially. It was while delivering a basket of Big Boys one day that Sam got on the subject of health. He said that the way he saw it, the Fountain of Youth was a watering can. He also said that maybe some people would do as well to push lawn mowers around as to ride bikes that don't go anywhere.

Ah, that Sam. His toil certainly hadn't tired his sense of humor.

I asked Sam that afternoon how he would rate his own level of fitness if he had to, and his answer didn't surprise me. He said he wasn't even sure what fitness was, but if it was what you got when you did "all the stuff" he saw me doing, he was pretty sure he didn't want any.

I couldn't let Sam leave that day without telling him that fitness like his was precisely what fitness like mine was hoping for.

I've relaxed my exercise habits considerably in recent years, and especially since getting involved in this book. I must confess, however, that I have not—like Dr. Stamford—been able to quit cold turkey. Maybe that's because my addiction has been more severe than Bryant's, or maybe it's because I simply lack his strength of will. But I can tell you this from the bottom of my athlete's heart: I wouldn't do it all over again even if I could live longer than Sam Petersen. When I had marathon fever in my early thirties, I would train carrying 10-pound dumbbells, wearing a rubber sweat suit and ski cap—in July. The amount of energy I have wasted over the past twenty years pursuing nothing more worthwhile than exhaustion is exhausting to think about. I could have raised enough tomatoes to feed half the state of Pennsylvania.

But that's sweat over the dam. I'll be wallowing in it for your benefit a little more later in this book, but the point we want to make here—and it's one that has been very instrumental in my own exercise slowdown—is simply that strenuous exercise is *not* the great health savior that the fitness movement's apostles have wanted us to believe. It can do precious little to counteract the effects of a bad diet, it has very little effect on lowering cholesterol or blood pressure, and it's no better than *mild* activity for purposes of weight loss. And yes, it can be downright dangerous for people with unhealthy hearts. Add the psychological burdens that a heavy exercise program can impose, and it's clear that the credo of "no pain, no gain" needs some reshaping of its own.

But if that's true—if strenuous exercise is *not* the periodic "spanking" that the human anatomy needs to keep in line—where did it get its reputation for being such a health enhancer in the first place?

That's an excellent question, the answer to which is central to the understanding of this book. Exercise has gotten its golden reputation largely through association. When people exercise, they also tend to lose weight, eat better, and cut back on vices, and these are the factors that have the far greater impact on their health. At the root of the fitness movement has been the premise that the heart needs to be worked hard in order to work well, but it's a supposition that has never been clinically proven. Yes, habitual strenuous exercise can strengthen the heart's ability to pump blood, but it's still very much in doubt whether that strength translates into protection from coronary artery disease, a condition in which the arteries that feed the heart become clogged with fatty deposits.

What strengthens the pump does not necessarily maintain the cleanliness of the pipes, in other words. The fatal heart attacks of 10-mile-a-day runner Jim Fixx and Olympic rower Jack Kelly made this point all too well. These men, highly fit though they were, had massive blocks in their coronary arteries that their daily workouts obviously had done fatally little to prevent.

But isn't it standard advice to take up aerobic exercise to lower serum cholesterol, the demon that blocks coronary arteries in the first place?

Yes, but aerobic exercise has been overrated as a means of accomplishing this. We've been led to believe that exercise causes a drop in serum cholesterol—the bad LDL type especially—but people who exercise but don't lose weight or change their diets rarely see any change in their LDL cholesterol at all. It's not uncommon, in fact, to find dangerously high levels of LDL cholesterol in highly fit endurance athletes with diets high in saturated fat. What exercise *can* do is raise HDL cholesterol, the good type believed to keep arteries clean, but the increase is small and takes considerable time and effort to achieve. Nor does increasing HDL cholesterol offset the bad effects of an elevated LDL, which tends to be diet related.

What about exercise for lowering blood pressure?

Again, exercise that results in weight loss usually is accompanied by a decrease in blood pressure, but exercise without weight loss demonstrates only modest effects.

Credit Where Credit Has Not Been Due

But if all this is true—if aerobic exercise is not the great health enhancer that the aerobic movement has led us to believe—how did the aerobic concept capture such scientific attention in the first place?

The answer is that *not enough attention was paid*. Not one of the fitness studies responsible for giving aerobic exercise its good name actually looked at aerobic exercise. Participants didn't jog, cycle, swim, or cross-country ski their way to better health. The studies looked at *moderate physical activity*, the kinds of activities people encounter in their leisure time and their jobs. These studies all arrived at the same conclusion: that, yes, a certain level of physical activity was necessary for avoiding undue risks of heart disease and other health problems. *None* of the studies, however, ever examined activity levels capable of producing aerobic fitness. The famed "British Transport Worker" study done in 1953, for example, found that ticket-takers on England's double-decker buses experienced lower rates of heart disease than the more sedentary drivers of these buses.

But were the ticket takers "aerobically fit"?

Very unlikely, given the fact that the only exercise they got was the standing, walking, and periodic stair-climbing they did on the job—certainly not fitness-producing activities by aerobic standards. And yet the aerobic movement interpreted the findings of this study as support for its aerobic fitness argument.

Then came the "San Francisco Longshoreman" study done in this country. Dock workers who engaged in loading activities were found to suffer less from heart disease than sedentary workers.

A case for aerobic fitness?

Given the intermittent nature of the activity of a dock worker, probably not, and yet results of the study, as with the British study, became fuel for the aerobics fire.

Other studies came along to fan the aerobic flame—studies of U.S. and Italian railroad workers, American farmers, British civil servants, kibbutz workers in Israel, Masai tribesmen, and Eskimos. And yes, the verdict of all these studies was that moderate physical activity seemed to be protective against heart disease. Aerobic exercise, however, the kind strenuous enough to sustain a substantially elevated heart rate for at least twenty minutes at a stretch, *had never even been considered* by these investigations.

That wasn't going to stop the aerobic forefathers from getting us out on the jogging trail, however. If some exercise was good, more was going to be better, and evidence to the contrary was not going to get discussed. Ignored, for example, was a 1966 study involving 110,000 people published in the *Journal of the American Medical Association*, which found that considerable heart disease protection was enjoyed by people who engaged in nothing more strenuous than recreational sporting activities or walking. Additional physical activity was found to offer little additional protection. The findings of that study speak for themselves:

Age-Adjusted Rates for Nonsmoking Men
(per 1,000 per year)

	Number of first heart attacks	% dying from first heart attack	Deaths within first 4 weeks
Least Active Men	5.2	56	2.9
Intermediate	2.9	18	0.5
Most Active Men	2.2	15	0.3

There was a sharp break between the least active and intermediate groups for nonfatal and fatal first heart attacks, but there was little difference between the intermediate and most active groups. The authors suggested that "a substantial reduction in mortality might be achieved through a relatively small increase in habitual physical activities of the most inactive men in a given population."

Source: JAMA 198(12):1241–1245, 1966: Copyright 1966, American Medical Association.

You don't have to be highly active, in other words, in order to gain considerable protection from our number one killer, but the aerobic founders wanted us pounding the pavements anyway. Dr. Ken Cooper's best-selling book, *Aerobics*, marked the official launch of the aerobics movement in 1968, and the era of "you get what you sweat for" had been born.

Born, but never scientifically verified. Millions of Americans began training for marathons believing that, as Dr. Thomas Bassler proclaimed, anyone who could run 26.2 miles would be *immune* to heart disease. The fitness craze quickly generated a considerable amount of commercial momentum, and the movement was soon off and running with such speed that no one stopped to question whether it really had a leg to stand on. Not until recently, in fact, some twenty years later, has research begun to examine the "no pain, no gain" and "more is better" philosophies from a scientific standpoint. On the surface, these philosophies had always seemed to make sense, and they certainly fit well with the nose-to-the-grindstone work ethnic we've always thought to be at the heart of American greatness. But would they hold up under a second round of close scientific inspection?

No, they would not. Some exercise is necessary for health—that message has held up. But once you get up and about and move beyond the couch potato stage, increased amounts of exercise pay only minor additional dividends. As much as that seems to fly in the face of everything the fitness movement has stood for, the argument has some very convincing evidence on its side. For starters, there are the studies by Dr. Ralph Paffenbarger and Dr. Arthur Leon, which were discussed earlier. There are others as well. For example:

□ A study of 3,975 Finnish men reported that leisure-time physical activity levels of 2,000 calories a week were found to afford as much protection from heart disease as activity levels far in excess of that. This finding agrees perfectly with the findings of the Harvard alumni study conducted by Dr. Paffenbarger. The authors recommend a daily energy expenditure of 200 to 300 calories as a means of substantially improving the health of sedentary individuals. (See *European Heart Journal* 8:1047–1055, 1987.)

□ A 1989 study of 13,344 men and women by researchers at the Institute for Aerobics Research in Dallas is the largest study of its kind ever conducted. The findings created headlines in the *New York Times*, *Newsweek*, *Time*, and *USA Today* and were discussed on a number of television programs. The study showed that: (1) having a low level of fitness "is an important risk factor for all-cause mortality in both men and women" (being a couch potato is dangerous to your health, in other words); (2) modest amounts of exercise can markedly reduce the risks of heart disease and cancer of the colon; and (3) a high fitness level doesn't offer more protection against heart disease than a moderate fitness level. Walking 30 to 60 minutes a day, say the authors, is a good example of the kind of exercise needed to maximize health benefits. "This is a hopeful message, an important message for the American people to understand," said Dr. Carl Caspersen of the Centers for Disease Control in Atlanta in an interview with the *New York Times*. "You don't have to be a marathoner. In fact, you get much more benefit out of being just a bit more active" (Journal of the American Medical Association 262 (1989) 2395–2401).*

The verdict at last seems clear: All other things being equal, the gardener's odds against heart disease are as good as the marathoner's. Moderate levels of activity can keep the cardiovascular system as healthy as extreme levels of activity. The credo of "no pain, no gain" has been all wet with its own sweat.

Please note: Large-scale epidemiological studies—the kind discussed in this book—control carefully, with the aid of sophisticated statistical techniques, the potential influence of confounding factors such as cigarette smoking, high blood pressure, and obesity. In other words, the physically active individuals in these studies do not demonstrate more protection from heart disease than their sedentary counterparts simply because they have better health habits. Physical activity, in and of itself and independent from other factors, offers the protection.

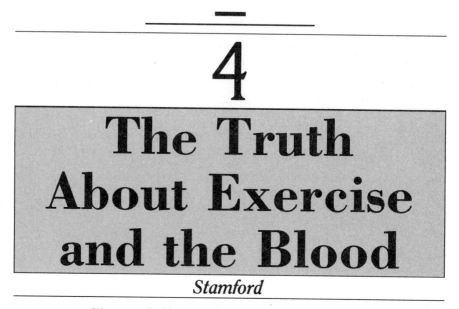

4

The Truth About Exercise and the Blood

Stamford

Weary and old . . . to the mercy of a rude stream.
—William Shakespeare, 1564–1616

So the aerobic apostles have been asking for a pound of flesh when just a few ounces will do. They've also been pinching at the fat on our hips and thighs, and checking our pulses, and wanting to know how long we can hold up on a treadmill.

Are these really the best ways to measure health?

No, they are not. They're good ways to measure aerobic fitness—the body's ability to perform oxygen-consuming exercise for extended periods of time—but they are not reliable indicators of overall health. Some very fit people, as we've seen, have died at an early age. A better way to measure overall health, and especially one's odds against heart disease, is to test the blood. Without fit blood, a fit heart is a goner even if it is in the chest of a marathoner. Let's see why.

The blood is amazing and important stuff. It manages to deliver not just oxygen to virtually every cell in the body, but food, water, first-aid in the form of germ-fighting compounds, even "moral support" in the form of hormones capable of regulating everything from happiness to sex drive. The blood is the body's keeper, and it's especially responsible for avoiding heart disease.

When I try to explain this to people in my health promotion classes, they often seem confused. They think of heart disease as a problem with the heart, not the blood. But it's not so. Most heart attacks occur in people whose hearts are actually clinically healthy. The cause of these heart attacks is a shortage of oxygen to the heart muscle—the result of arteries leading to the heart becoming blocked because of unfit blood.

What lets blood get "out of shape"?

It's not lack of exercise. It's not a lack of anything, for that matter. It's a surplus of things:

- Too much saturated fat in the diet, which can cause the liver to infuse the blood with too much artery-clogging LDL cholesterol, and also raise blood pressure
- Too much stress in the lifestyle, which can cause the adrenal glands to pollute the blood with too much artery-damaging and cholesterol-raising adrenaline
- Too much carbon monoxide, if you're a smoker, which can reduce the ability of the blood to carry oxygen, and hence damage arteries by slowly "suffocating" the cells that make up their interior walls.

It's a multiphased process that finally stops the heart, but it all comes back to blood "unfit" for coronary consumption.

How can blood be kept in shape?

That's what this book is about. You can engage in regular aerobic exercise, which will have only very minor effects, or you can eat the right diet and get a handle on stress and smoking, which will have very major effects. Let's take a quick journey through the bloodstream as well as the scientific literature to see why this is true.

Your Heart's Best Friend Is Your Mouth

Sorry, fitness buffs, but exercise—no matter how hard or how long—has no impact on LDL cholesterol, the kind that shows the greatest tendency to collect inside artery walls.

The reason?

LDL cholesterol is not a fuel. Your muscles don't burn it like carbohydrates or fats. The only thing aerobic exercise does is propel LDL cholesterol through the arteries at an accelerated pace.

Diet is what affects LDL cholesterol, and that's why we'll be emphasizing the importance of what you eat in the pages ahead more than the amount of aerobic exercise you perform. Your mouth can protect you from heart disease more than your muscles. We've said it before and we'll be saying it again: By reducing the saturated fat in your diet, you slow your liver's output of LDL cholesterol. Aerobic exercise will have no such effect.

But wait. Doesn't aerobic exercise boost HDL cholesterol, the "good" kind that tends to keep LDL cholesterol from getting into artery-clogging trouble in the first place?

Yes, but it takes more than just a few jumping jacks to build those HDLs. Marathon runners and other highly fit endurance athletes who engage regularly in huge amounts of aerobic exercise can reach unusually high HDL levels, but to assume that the same will hold true for the novice jogger or three-times-a-week aerobic dancers is a gross misinterpretation of the evidence. The following studies make this quite clear.

□ A 1982 study in the *Journal of the American Medical Association* by Williams and colleagues from Stanford University found that men who ran at least 10 miles a week for nine months experienced HDL increases that could be considered modest, at best. Those who ran less than 10 miles a week, moreover, saw negligible improvement, and the improvement in the two groups overall was less than 2 mg./dl.—not a great payoff for nine months work.

□ A 1988 study in the medical journal *Circulation* by Paul Thompson and colleagues from Brown University found that men pushed "to the subjective limits of their training capacity" in exercise sessions lasting an hour each, five days a week for eight to twelve months, experienced HDL increases of only about 5 mg./dl.—again, not a lot of gain for the pain.

Other studies report similar modest gains in HDL despite considerable effort, and short-term studies lasting less than twenty weeks generally report no change. This notoriously had been the case with the fitness classes I used to conduct that lasted ten weeks. Little or no change would result, regardless of how hard people worked.

Does this mean we write high HDLs off for all but the most dedicated fitness fanatics?

Not necessarily. Some evidence does suggest that moderate physical activity, such as walking, can boost HDL levels somewhat if done over a long enough period of time. Postal carriers in a study by researchers from the University of Pittsburgh's Department of Epidemiology, for example, were found to have higher than average HDLs. Habitual activity may have an effect, even though a modest one. Considering, too, that people who get virtually no exercise—especially those who are confined to power-driven wheelchairs—show dangerously low HDL levels, and the argument for moderate activity looks even stronger. The research leaves little doubt that the greatest health benefits stand to be gained by people willing simply to raise their activity levels beyond a totally sedentary state.

Getting the HDLs "Up" by Getting the LDLs Down

But the argument for raising HDLs through aerobic exercise becomes almost meaningless, considering the effect that diet can have on blood cholesterol. HDLs are the blood's scavengers, their job being to keep LDLs from reaching such high concentrations that they begin infiltrating artery walls. But by keeping LDLs low, through diet, you reduce the need for high HDLs in the first place. This is why such attention is now given to what you may have heard about as the "total cholesterol/HDL ratio." What the ratio indicates is whether or not your HDLs are in the company of more LDLs than they can handle. If your ratio is low—less than about 3.5 to 1—your risks for heart disease are low because your HDLs are not being seriously outnumbered. But if your ratio is high—more than about 5 to 1—you could be in trouble. The average American man has this 5 to 1 ratio, which is one reason why rates of heart disease in the United States remain so high. The average ratio among American women is 4.5 to 1—better, and probably one of the reasons women's odds against heart disease are better. A ratio of 4.5 to 1, however, is still too high for optimum coronary comfort.

To get a better idea of just how diet and exercise compare in this all-important matter of improving blood "fitness," let's look at some numbers. If you were to jog faithfully for an hour a day, five days a week for one year, you might expect your HDLs to climb by about 5 mg./dl.—the increase experienced by the participants in Dr. Thompson's study cited above.

What would this do to your all-important total cholesterol/HDL ratio?

Assuming your blood was "average" for adult men (215 total cholesterol, 43 HDL) at the start of the jogging program, the 5 mg./dl. increase would drop your ratio by about half a point—from 5 to 1 to 4.5 to 1.

Worth the year of sweat?

If you enjoyed the running, yes. But if you didn't, you'd certainly have to wonder if there might not have been an easier way.

Now let's look at me. When I was running 30 miles a week, plus lifting weights in my heyday, I had a ratio—are you ready for this?—of 6.2 to 1.

And now? Thanks to my far more sensible diet, 3.5 to 1. I have cut my risks of heart disease from greater than average to less than half the average despite abandoning aerobic exercise.

But aren't I going to be missing those few extra HDLs I had when I was exercising aerobically?

Research suggests not, because as we've seen, high HDL levels appear to be important only if LDL levels are also high. Fewer criminals require fewer police. It's a phenomenon illustrated best of all, perhaps, by the famed Tarahumara Indians of Mexico. Despite the incredible 100-mile weeks of running these people manage to fit into their lifestyles, their average HDL level is a surprisingly low 27 mg./dl.—a good 15 points lower than the average American couch potato.

Heart disease among the Tarahumaras?

Almost nonexistent because of their extremely low-fat diets. The Tarahumaras get only about 10 percent of their calories from fat, which keeps their total cholesterol—and hence LDLs—extremely low.

The Tarahumaras have led some researchers to speculate that only in societies such as ours, where fat intake is high, does aerobic exercise result in HDL increases. HDL police may rise to the occasion, in other words, only if there's enough LDL trouble in the streets (bloodstream) to warrant their services. A diet low in fat may keep enough LDL "peace" so that large numbers of HDLs are not needed.

Know Where You Stand

The latest guidelines issued by the National Institutes of Health (NIH) are calling for total cholesterol levels below 200. "High" risk of heart disease, they say, begins at about 240. More than half of the adults in the United States have cholesterol levels above the desirable range (200 mg./dl.), and half of these have values above 240.

How do you measure up?

If you do not yet know your cholesterol numbers, you are in the majority. According to a 1986 survey, only about half of American adults had ever had their cholesterol measured, and only about 7 percent knew their numbers. I'm certain these statistics have improved since 1987, when the new guidelines were introduced, but we still have a long way to go. If you haven't had your cholesterol checked, do so. And if it's above 200, pay attention to the dietary advice we'll be giving later in this book.

Is there a cholesterol level that could be low enough to make fatty buildup in the arteries virtually impossible?

That's a tough question to answer, because rarely does cholesterol work in isolation. Its effects can be greatly magnified by cigarette smoking, high blood pressure, and stress. Do consider this, however. Data from the over forty-plus-year history of the world famous Framingham Heart Study indicate that the risk of heart attack begins to rise at levels of 140 to 150, and then shoots up dramatically beyond 200. This suggests that a cholesterol level below 150 is a strong defense against heart disease.

But whether or not you are successful in lowering your cholesterol to below 150, you will reap dividends from just lowering it. The Lipid

Research Clinics Coronary Primary Prevention Trial followed 3,806 men with dangerously elevated cholesterol levels for up to ten years. Those who successfully reduced their cholesterol reduced their risk of heart attack. For every 1 percent drop in cholesterol, their risk of heart disease dropped 2 percent. Results of the study make a strong argument for giving your cholesterol level a serious look.

A Word on Cholesterol and Cancer

Get your cholesterol under 200 mg./dl. as a first step, then feel free to go lower. And do not worry about rumors that low cholesterol can be a risk for cancer. Yes, some studies have found a relationship between cancer of the bowel and a very low blood cholesterol level, but there's no evidence that the low cholesterol caused the cancer. And there's certainly no evidence to support that a low cholesterol brought about by a diet low in saturated fat is associated with cancer of the bowel.

The association that was reported in a few studies, but not in others, is more likely due to the fact that cancer of the colon may cause a drop in cholesterol. In a similar way, people who have their gall bladders removed often have low cholesterol because they can't store bile and the body has to use much of its cholesterol to constantly make new bile supplies. Had their low cholesterol levels caused them to lose their gall bladders? Of course not.

What's more, if low blood cholesterol caused cancer of the bowel, there would be an epidemic in many foreign countries where low cholesterol levels are the norm. But in such countries, cancer of the bowel is rare. It's far more common in the United States, in fact, where cholesterol levels are high. There's no reason to fear a low cholesterol level as long as you eat the type of nutritious diet that we recommend in this book.

Alcohol Not So Cordial

How does the new cholesterol research impact on the supposed HDL-raising and hence heart-friendly effects of alcohol?

Hold the next round. Drinking to help prevent heart disease has been an understandably popular notion over the years, and although alcohol seems to raise HDL, there may not be a corresponding decrease in heart disease risk. HDL has subfractions called HDL2 and HDL3. HDL2 appears to be the heart helper, while HDL3 is neutral. Marathon running can increase HDL2, but there is no evidence that alcohol exerts the same beneficial effects. Therefore, all things considered, alcohol would have to be viewed as less of a friend to the heart than a foe. It can encourage obesity because of its empty calories, it can raise blood pressure, and it can elevate triglycerides (another blood fat suspected of contributing to heart attack). We'll be talking more about alcohol and some other vices in Part IV, but keep in mind for now that the stuff needs to be treated with respect for the cardiovascular party-pooper it can be.

Heart Disease Under the Microscope

This chapter would not be complete without a description of how heart attacks actually occur. It's important that you understand the nature of the beast that stalks and kills more than 500,000 Americans every year. Learn all you can, and apply it.

The heart is a miraculous muscle. It's only about as big as your fist and weighs less than a pound, but it has the strength to move blood through thousands of miles of blood vessels with every beat.

And what does the heart ask for in return for such amazing service?

One thing more than anything else: oxygen. A constant supply of oxygen is so important to the heart that the arteries responsible for the job are massive in relation to the heart itself. It's as though it was anticipated from the very beginning that we might someday be clogging these arteries with the likes of double-bacon cheeseburgers.

When the coronary arteries become blocked to the point that they cannot carry enough oxygen-rich blood to the heart, several things can happen. Heart muscle can begin to die gradually, the result being a condition known as congestive heart failure, in which the heart becomes dangerously enlarged from incoming blood, which it lacks the strength to pump. Eventually the heart "drowns" in this excess blood and stops altogether.

More common, however, is the heart attack that strikes quickly. Narrowed coronary arteries offer a sticking point for blood clots, called thrombi, which can stop blood flow suddenly and fatally. But even though the atherosclerotic (clogging) process is ongoing, and even though the arteries may become dangerously narrow, there are no symptoms. Only when the clogging process has reached alarming proportions—70 to 80 percent closure—does the heart begin to ache, and by then it may be too late to head off an attack.

And how exactly do blood vessels become narrowed in the first place? And can blockage be reversed?

The primary culprit is believed to be LDL cholesterol, the trouble-maker that the liver produces in response to a diet too rich in saturated fat. And yes, there is growing evidence that arterial clogging can be reversed to some degree, as we'll be seeing shortly.

Some LDL cholesterol is necessary for hormone and cell production, and it can enter the cells of artery walls in limited amounts through specialized LDL receptors. But too much LDL in the blood can trigger infiltration of artery walls in mass, and the process is made worse by high blood pressure, which creates tiny lesions (wounds) through which LDLs can enter the arterial lining. Once inside, LDLs become trapped, bulging as they accumulate, eventually impinging on the flow of blood.

This is why doctors consider lowering blood pressure and lowering serum cholesterol to be of equal and such utmost importance in heart disease prevention. The two make a very dangerous duo. Add smoking and a lot of emotional stress and you go from dangerous to deadly. Smoking ranks so high as a heart disease risk factor not so much because of nicotine, but because of carbon monoxide. The carbon monoxide in cigarette smoke attaches to circulating red blood cells in place of oxygen, the result being not just trouble for the heart directly, but trouble for the cells that make up artery walls. They weaken without adequate oxygen, thus making the LDL invasion even easier. Emotional stress promotes LDL production, which adds fuel to the fire.

When I present this scenario of "blood vessel vandalism" caused by high cholesterol, hypertension, smoking, and negative stress, people understandably express concern, especially the smokers and loyal patrons of fast-food restaurants. They want to know how they can get the health of their vascular networks checked out.

My answer?

Vow to change the behavior that's worrying you, and then make an appointment for a good physical. The only way to assess the cleanliness of the arteries directly is by way of a very expensive and somewhat dangerous technique that threads a tube, starting usually at an incision made at the thigh, clear up to the heart. "Ouch" is right.

Simply by getting a good physical, on the other hand, your doctor should be able to make a good guess at what sort of shape your blood vessels are in. If your blood is "unfit" and driven with high pressure, or you're under a lot of stress and you smoke, you've pretty much got your answer. Make changes now!

And if there is already considerable clogging?

Be assured that in all of us there will be some clogging, even in the offspring of the offspring of baby boomers. As early as 1915, scientists called attention to the childhood origin of atherosclerosis, and autopsies performed on young American soldiers killed in Korea and Vietnam showed advanced clogging in a significant percentage. Atherosclerosis may begin at birth, progressing with age and becoming clinically significant in mid to late life—the rate of progress is dictated by lifestyle and genetic predisposition.

But don't despair. Better late than never. The fact that you don't have symptoms such as chest pain (angina pectoris) suggests that the process has not reached the critical stage. Arrest the process now with the lipofitness lifestyle, and chances are good that you can live comfortably and well with whatever arterial clearance you have left.

Any chance of unclogging?

Intriguing new research suggests that arterial blockage can actually be reversed. The key seems to be the type of diet we recommend in this book—one very low in saturated fat. This, combined with the kind of moderate daily exercise we also recommend and avoidance of smoking and negative stress, appears capable of gradually clearing arteries of plaque buildup. Pioneering the research in this area has been San Francisco cardiologist Dr. Dean Ornish. Preliminary results from his research look promising, and results from other studies also offer reason for optimism.

So do not despair over past sins. Atherosclerosis appears to be a disease which can be stopped and possibly even persuaded to make a U-turn.

Fit but Not Healthy: The Case of John

We would like to close this chapter by again affirming that we are not opposed to aerobic exercise, nor are we saying that aerobic exercise can't have some effect in reducing heart disease risks. But we are saying that when the effect of an aerobic exercise program is compared with that of a low-saturated-fat diet, there's no contest—exercise loses badly. A combination of both is fine, but only if you enjoy the exercise. If exercise is punishment, forget it, and your odds against heart disease will not suffer as long as you cover all the other dietary and stress-control bases. There can be danger, in fact, in putting too much faith in the protective powers of a rigorous exercise program. Consider the case of John.

Tan, lean, muscular, John had come to my Fitness Evaluation Center at the University of Louisville for a cardiovascular stress test at the insistence of his wife. As far as John was concerned, however, he was on his way to living to be a hundred, and he had reasons for believing so. His morning jogs and six hours a week of intensely competitive singles tennis had him looking a lot younger than his fifty-four years. But it didn't take long for me to see why John's wife was afraid that his health might only be skin deep. He was as ornery as a wounded badger, wanting to know nothing more than how long the test was going to take.

Well, it didn't take very long, as it turned out, because once he was on the treadmill it became clear very quickly that John's heart was having significant difficulty receiving sufficient blood through his coronary arteries. The attending cardiologist terminated the test, and a heated discussion ensued. John refused to believe that he could have a problem, given his athletic lifestyle and physique. He went so far as to accuse the cardiologist of being incompetent. Our only recourse was to suggest to John that he seek a second opinion, which he did. He underwent a cardiac catheterization, which revealed advanced blockage in two of the three major arteries of his heart and a moderate blockage in the third. John underwent bypass surgery several weeks later.

The moral of John's story?

Don't look to a lean physique that's been sculpted by strenuous exercise as a guarantee of good health. John's diet, his wife later told us, was atrociously high in fat, and his personality, as we learned first hand, was akin to a time bomb. John's exercise was doing as poor a job of counteracting his diet as it was of moderating his high-strung personality—yet further evidence that the human heart lives not by exercise alone.

5

Calculations on Exercise and Longevity

Shimer

Grow old along with me
The best is yet to be
—Robert Browning, 1812–1889

Exercise doesn't make you live longer, it only makes it seem like you do."

You're likely to hear that one get a few chuckles at the local taproom or doughnut shop. But hang out at a health club or a local sporting goods store and you're apt to hear a very different tune.

"Use it or lose it. He who rests rusts."

Who's right here? Whether or not exercise can greatly reduce risks of heart disease, can it promote long life in other ways? Is exercise a lubricator of the body's longevity gears, in other words, or does it merely spin those gears, maybe even wear them out?

The argument has been going on since the Athenian messenger Pheidippides finished D.O.A. after his 26.2-mile run from the city of Marathon to Athens, Greece, in 400 B.C. Most prominent among the exercise bashers has been cardiologist Henry Solomon, M.D., whose best-seller *The Exercise Myth* in 1984 had people strapping themselves to their easy chairs. Before that, as you'll recall from "The Case of the Dangling Heart" in chapter 2, J. E. Schmidt, M.D., claimed jogging impacted on the body with enough force to turn the internal organs to mush.

Such hyperbole on the part of the prosecution, however, has not been unmatched by the defense. Thomas Bassler, M.D., gained widespread recognition for his claim that the ability to run a marathon guaranteed immunity from heart disease, no questions asked. And an army of eager young exercise physiologists encouraged the masses to jog, row, cycle, or swim their way to everlasting health.

You can see that the exercise/longevity issue has been a heated one. Data have been gathered in the past few years, however, that should ice the issue down somewhat. What the new data suggest is that an active lifestyle can extend lifespan by approximately . . .

On second thought, we think we'll make you guess. The question boils down to this: Person A leads an active lifestyle from the age of about twenty years on, while Person B does not. Assuming their lifestyles are identical in all other ways, will Person A outlive Person B, and if so, by how much?

a. Person A will not necessarily outlive Person B.
b. Person A will outlive Person B by about two years.
c. Person A will outlive Person B by about four years.
d. Person A will outlive Person B by about eight years.
e. Person A will outlive Person B by about eleven years.

Dr. Stamford and I conducted a little survey of our own regarding this question, and it surprised us that inactive people tended to make higher guesses than active people. Many of the active people remarked that _quality_ of life was more important to them than quantity, and by quality they meant keeping their weight under control and relieving stress. Inactive people, on the other hand, tended to express feelings of guilt for their inactivity, though we did confront our share of couch potatoes who must have been fans of the early works of J. E. Schmidt.

So what's the answer?

The answer is "b"—an active person will outlive an inactive person by an average of about two years. If that depresses you, the following bit of arithmetic might depress you even more. In response to the _New England Journal of Medicine_ study that offered the figure of two years, a cardiologist from the University of California at San Francisco wrote to that journal with some calculations of his own. The doctor, David B. Jacoby, M.D., of the Cardiovascular Research Institute at UCSF, had determined that depending on exercise intensity, the amount of time it would take to do the amount of exercise needed to extend life by two years would come to . . .

Two years! "Thus, the bad news is that although you may live an extra two years, those two years will be spent jogging," Dr. Jacoby wrote.

Not exactly wind for the old jogging sails, is it?

Or is it? We got to thinking about the seemingly absurd trade-off suggested by Dr. Jacoby's arithmetic, and it occurred to us that it's absurd only if what you do to gain those two years is unenjoyable or unproductive. If what you do is pleasurable or accomplishes something—even if it's just cutting the grass—then there's no absurdity, only great wisdom in those efforts. You're getting two years of pleasure and/or work done *plus* two years of future for having done so. What better deal than that? Only activities that are burdensome or unproductive qualify as absurd according to Dr. Jacoby's math. Pleasurable and purposeful activities make the two-year deal look like a very good one.

Every Step You Take

In the same issue of the *New England Journal of Medicine* in which Dr. Jacoby's letter appeared, two physicians from the Johns Hopkins University School of Medicine presented calculations that support the kind of exercise wisdom we're talking about. Drs. Brent Petty and David Herrington determined that the amount of exercise needed to earn the extra two years of life in question could be accomplished by *just six minutes a day of stair-climbing*. They calculated, in fact, that *four seconds of extra life could be gained for every step taken*.

Now, that's the kind of thinking that's going to provide the solution to this seemingly inescapable exercise dilemma so many of us claim to face. Not enough time? Not enough coordination? Not enough facilities?

You must live in the Gobi Desert if there are no stairs in your life. In addition to being a "time-effective method to increase longevity," Drs. Petty and Herrington called stair-climbing "an expedient method of getting from one floor to another."

We rest our case. Exercise opportunities are everywhere. We just need to open our eyes to them.

How Important the Genes?

But aren't we forgetting something? Aren't we forgetting that someone like George Burns can yuk it up into his nineties despite a halo of cigar smoke around his head and a love affair with the dry martini? Aren't we forgetting that Winston Churchill made it to ninety-one despite brandy for breakfast and a midsection that was world famous for being so "global"?

Compare these cases to the tragically early deaths of superbly conditioned professional football player Brian Piccolo of cancer, and legendary

New York Yankee first baseman Lou Gehrig. Does our fate get determined in the split second it takes sperm to meet egg? Are we puppets on chromosomal strings merely acting out the script that was written the day Dad's DNA collaborated with Mom's? We joke that good health boils down to choosing our parents wisely, but in light of the evidence maybe it's no joke. Should we put the tennis racquet and wheat germ aside and just let our genes run their course?

We wish we had the final word on this one, but we don't, because no one does. Most authorities agree that we are indeed subservient to genetic influences, but to what degree has been the question. Do the genes dictate or merely predispose? Are they captain of the ship or merely crewman?

Certainly not the last word, but at least a well-crafted guess was made in 1988 by the authors of a study that appeared in the *New England Journal of Medicine*. The study, directed by Dr. Thorkild Sorensen, of the University of Copenhagen, looked at the lives of 960 people who had been adopted at a very young age, most at infancy. The goal of the analysis was to see whether the diseases these adoptees eventually died of would compare more closely to the diseases that their real parents had succumbed to, or would there be a closer connection to the diseases that had claimed their foster parents? Would genes or would environment prove to exert the greater influence?

Results were surprising. Genes seemed to dominate for some diseases, but not others. And the diseases that showed the greatest genetic influence were *not* the ones you would expect. For example: Strong genetic influence seemed to prevail for infectious diseases—specifically pneumonia, tuberculosis, and bronchitis—and to some degree heart attacks and strokes. Genes did *not* seem to be the predominant factor with cancer, however. Not by a long shot. Adoptees proved to be five times more likely to die of cancer if a foster parent had died of the disease before the age of fifty than if a biological parent had succumbed.

Infectious diseases, which we commonly think of as being "caught" instead of inherited, proved to be strongly genetic. And cancer, which we usually think of as being largely genetic, proved to be primarily environmental. Heart attacks and strokes wound up falling somewhere in between, suggesting that influences come equally from genes and environment alike. How could the results be explained?

Regarding infectious diseases, genes may determine the strength of the immune system. The number of colds someone gets a year, in other words, may be due as much to heritage as hand-washing. As for cancer, current thinking suggests an interaction between environmental and genetic factors. Surprisingly, however, the greatest impact seems to come from the environment—smoking, diet, and occupational factors, for example.

This means that if you have a shaky family tree regarding cancer, do not despair. How *you* live *your* life is what should be of concern to you. Lifestyle, not blood lines, seems to be the far greater cancer factor.

Heart disease and strokes?

It would be nice if there were none in your history, but even if there are, lifestyle may be able to cancel out the influence. And as for infectious diseases such as pneumonia, tuberculosis, and bronchitis, isn't it nice to know that modern science is giving us a helping hand? If weak immunity is a genetic hand-me-down, as the study suggests, at least it's comforting to know that innoculations are now capable of doing what our genes may not be.

The bottom line: *Good health is not just in the genes*; it's also very much in how you wear those genes. You may be able to "wrinkle" a good set of genes with an unhealthy lifestyle, in other words, but you also may be able to "iron out" a bad set with a healthy approach to life.

But there's another message here, and perhaps an even more important one because it stands to benefit our children. By knowing our genetic tendencies, we can warn them of theirs. A family tree strung with heart attacks like so many pine cones should serve as reason to be extra careful in having your children avoid high-fat foods, obesity, and a couch potato lifestyle. A family history of cancer also should serve as reason for them to avoid fatty foods and, of course, smoking.

"Cultural transmission can be even stronger than genetic transmission," in this regard, says Roger R. Williams, M.D., of the Cardiovascular Genetics Research Clinic of the University of Utah. That's because a "bad" gene can be expected to be passed on to only half of all offspring, whereas a "bad" habit can be expected to affect all offspring.

Get the message? You may not be able to give your kids a perfect set of chromosomes, but you can give them a clean set of living habits, which may be an even more important contribution in the long run.

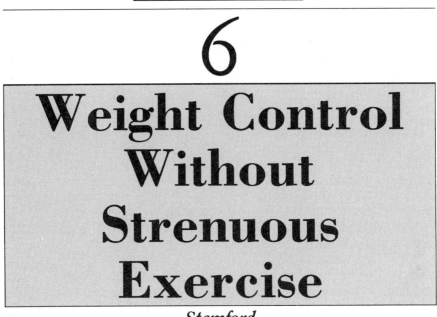

6

Weight Control Without Strenuous Exercise

Stamford

Little strokes fell great oaks.
—Benjamin Franklin, 1706–1790

But longevity aside, isn't aerobic exercise the best attack one can mount against body fat? Pick up any diet book, or at least any good diet book, and you'll learn how exercise can minimize the muscle loss associated with weight reduction and how it can elevate calorie-burning even at rest. You'll also learn how exercise can help control appetite and how it can give a psychological boost.

Are we going to tell you that all of these benefits have been made up by Jane Fonda's public relations team?

No, we are not. But we are going to tell you that you're being deceived if you think the kind of exercise needed to achieve those weight-loss advantages has to produce a "target heart rate" or that it even has to make you sweat. By laws of biochemistry as well as physics, calories burned by doing heavy activity count no more than those burned by doing light activity. Light activity may even be better for weight loss, in fact, if you're inclined to engage in it more frequently—after eating, especially, as we'll be seeing shortly.

What about exercises for specific areas of the body? Gardening can't trim saddlebags or flatten a pot belly, right?

True, but neither can specialized exercise programs. There's no such thing as "spot reduction"—reducing fact selectively from a specific body area, say the thighs or waist. When fat is burned as fuel it comes from storage depots all over the body, regardless of which muscles are active. The way to trim trouble spots is to trim down all over, and that's exactly what we plan to help you do—*without* monotonous and time-wasting exercises.

We could give you a lot of examples of people who successfully control their weight without strenuous exercise, but we decided to choose me because for more than twenty years heavy exercise was the *only* way I controlled my weight. From my teens through my late thirties, I exercised hard for at least forty-five minutes a day no fewer than five days a week. Between running and lifting weights, I was burning an average of about 500 calories per workout—for more than twenty years! You can imagine my fears when I decided to give it all up. I saw myself turning from Arnold Schwarzenegger to Rodney Dangerfield overnight, losing a good deal of respect along the way.

But it hasn't happened. It's been several years since I got off the exercise treadmill, and yet I now weigh even a little *less* than I did in my exercise heydays. My cholesterol also is lower—about 100 points lower, in fact—and I'm even trimmer in what had always been troublesome territory to me, that odious area of the "love handles."

As an exercise physiologist, how can I explain it?

Several factors have been responsible. Yes, the physical activity in my life is now very mild compared to what it used to be, but it's also *more frequent.* Whereas I used to compact all the physical activity in my life into intense forty-five-minute workouts and then do virtually nothing for the rest of the day, I now seize on all the opportunities for activity that I can, no matter how small. I've taught myself to think of calorie-burning in terms of a piggy bank as opposed to a safety deposit box. Every penny counts, and of course nickels and dimes count even more, but the point is that weight control doesn't have to rely on the kind of investments that can wind up leaving you feeling "broke" in terms of energy levels for anything else. In the old days, for example, my wife was lucky to get me to help unload grocery bags from the car once I had numbed myself with my aerobic fix. Now I'll offer to help, and I'll take the appropriate number of trips rather than endanger the goods by attempting four bags at once. No more eggs scrambled on the driveway. What I've done is to infiltrate my life with light, energizing, and useful activity rather than besiege it with exhausting and useless workouts. Let's walk through an average day to get a better idea of what I'm talking about.

Much of my work involves sitting at a desk with few interruptions—so I make interruptions. I'll get up at various times throughout the day and take off down the hall to find a flight of stairs. Once up, once down, and I'm on my way back to my desk. I call this a "mini-walk." If it's nice outside, I'll sometimes take what I call a "mini-walk plus," which means about a five-minute stroll down the block. I also look for reasons to walk—trips to the mailroom, for example, and other errands, as well. I come back refreshed, perky, and my low back feels better. I'm ready for another couple of rounds of whatever being sedentary has to dish out.

How many mini-walks do I take a day?

My real victory has been that I'm not even sure. I've cured myself of having to quantify the exercise in my life. I'm going to guess, however, that I might take anywhere from eight to twelve mini-walks a day. Assuming each is good for about 16 calories worth of energy expenditure (I try to include at least one flight of stairs in each walk), that comes to an average of 160 calories a day. It's not a lot compared to the 360 or so I used to burn on a 3-mile run, but the point is that I have been *energized* by these little bouts of physical activity rather than drained by them. When I get home I'm eager to get more activity rather than fall into a trance in front of the TV, as I used to do. A little trick has helped here, too. I make it a point to walk across the street to the hospital on my way to my car and walk up several flights of stairs. Now I'm perked up for my drive home, instead of merely hanging on at the end of the day. At home, off comes the tie, on go the blue jeans, and I'm either cutting grass, finding then carrying then stacking firewood, planting or pruning trees, doing routine house chores, having fun playing with the dog, or walking with my wife.

Weekends?

No more 10-milers that would wash me out for the rest of the day. I'll go for a hike in the woods, take a bike ride, go on a canoe trip, walk the dog, wash the car, or even just go shopping. The point is that I try to keep moving, and preferably in ways that are as enjoyable as possible. No more "empty calories" spent pursuing nothing more profitable than fatigue.

On Sundays, my grown sons visit and we toss barbells around in the garage. I really look forward to pumping a little iron, but the key is that I'm not "working" at it. It's play, and it's fun—a kind of flashback to being a kid again. And how much I lift and for how many reps is not a concern—it can't be if it's to continue being fun. I never thought I could feel this way about exercise, especially lifting weights.

Four Rounds Rather Than Three Squares

The bottom line is that I'm probably averaging about 300 calories of physical activity a day and hence about 2,100 for the week, enough to satisfy the 2,000 figure that Dr. Paffenbarger's research (see chapter 1) suggests affords substantial protection against heart disease. It's less than what I had been getting, but two other factors are now at play that are more than making up for the difference. One of those factors is the greater number of *smaller* meals that I'm eating, and the other is the low-fat composition of those meals.

When I was on my one-grueling-workout-a-day routine, I had to be careful to have at least three hours between when I would eat and when I would exercise. Severe indigestion would result if I didn't, and sometimes worse. The eating pattern that this forced me into was not a good one: I'd get most of my calories in one gluttonous sitting at night. As we'll be seeing later in this book, that's the worst way to eat for anyone trying to reduce body fat. Large meals call up large amounts of insulin, and insulin encourages calories to be stored as fat rather than burned. Worse yet, large meals tend to leave one feeling drowsy, and hence uninclined to do much more than sink into the nearest sofa, as I can attest to all too well.

Now, however, because the physical activity I do is very light, I can eat as frequently as I want, which is usually about four or five times a day. I'll have my usual good-size oatmeal and banana breakfast, a small midmorning snack of fruit, skim milk, or cottage cheese, a small lunch, an afternoon snack (usually on the weekends), and a decent but not in-decent-size dinner. It adds up to the same number of calories I used to eat in my heavy exercise days, but because the calories are much lower in fat, they're not demonstrating the same proclivity for sticking to my ribs, and I mean that quite literally.

New research is showing that calories from fat are considerably more likely to convert to body fat than calories from carbohydrates or protein. It's a point we'll be making repeatedly in this book as one of the major pillars of our *Fitness Without Exercise* platform. *Most body fat starts as dietary fat.* Say it out loud, if you think it'll help.

By keeping moderately active throughout the day—instead of being intensively active and then comatose—I have been able to benefit from a physiological phenomenon known as the Thermic Effect of Food (TEF). Research shows that the body's metabolic rate goes up by about 10 percent after a meal as a result of the processes it takes to get that meal digested. This 10 percent can be almost *doubled*, however, if light physical activity is pursued as those digestive processes are still going on. We'll be dis-cussing the TEF phenomenon in greater detail in Part III, but hold this analogy in your mind for the time being: It helps to fan a fire the minute you put on the wood. By pulling oxygen into the body within thirty minutes of eating, food can be made to burn hotter, in a sense, with fewer calories being available for fat storage as a result. This isn't to suggest you should follow Thanksgiving dinner with a marathon, but it does point to the advantages of light activity such as walking or yardwork within about a half hour of eating moderately. An added advantage is that having something to do after meals tends to keep meals from dragging on. It's tough to pick at leftovers, after all, if you're in the back yard playing a game of croquet.

Exercise Versus Activity: The Numbers Don't Lie

But can such a casual approach to weight loss really work?

Absolutely. Consider the case of Diane, a forty-three-year-old school teacher and mother of two who tried unsuccessfully for a year to lose weight by attending a low-impact aerobics class twice a week. She enjoyed the classes once she got there, but getting there was a problem, so when she asked me for advice I suggested she skip the classes and—like me—simply be more active. She loved to garden and play golf, and she always wanted to try horseback riding, so we put together the following program. As you can see, she now burns a lot more calories in a week than she used to with her aerobics class. She has also finally begun to lose weight. (For a more complete list of the calories* burned by activities less strenuous than aerobic exercise, see chapter 12.)

DIANE'S "AEROBIC" EFFORT

		Calories burned
Monday	off	—
Tuesday	45 minutes of aerobics	200
Wednesday	off	—
Thursday	45 minutes of aerobics	200
Friday	off	—
Saturday	30 minutes of stationary cycling	180
Sunday	off	—
Total calories burned:		**580**

DIANE'S "ACTIVITY" EFFORT

		Calories burned
Monday	30 minutes of gardening (digging)	200
Tuesday	30 minutes of walking	120
Wednesday	30 minutes of badminton	170
Thursday	30 minutes of walking	120
Friday	30 minutes of gardening (weeding)	130
Saturday	60 minutes of horseback riding	145
Sunday	9 holes of golf, pulling club carrier	180
Total calories burned:		**1,065**

Please note: The units are actually in kilocalories (Kcals). We use the word "calories" throughout because it is familiar and allows easy interpretation.

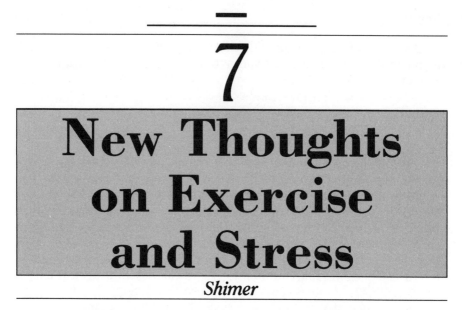

7

New Thoughts on Exercise and Stress

Shimer

It is characteristic of wisdom not to do desperate things.
—Henry David Thoreau, 1817–1862

Yet another claim made by the aerobic crusaders is that adherence to a regular aerobic exercise program can help combat psychological stress. The argument is that strenuous exercise can help the body "burn off" stress-induced hormones while at the same time helping to build a more positive and hence stress-resistant self-image.

And for some, this is no doubt true. People who have a regular exercise program that they feel comfortable with can rely on the program both as a release and a spirit-lifter.

But, what about the millions of us for whom exercise constitutes a stress: Rita, for example, who shoulders the guilt of having dropped out of at least one exercise class a year since 1982? Or Jean, who has managed to stick with her exercise class but hates it, and also hates the pinch that it puts on her time. Is that stress control?

Or how about Steve, who gets so worked up by his lunch hour squash matches that he has to have two beers to calm down? Or Bob, a dedicated marathon runner who nearly goes crazy every time he's sidelined with an injury? Has exercise constituted effective stress control for these individuals?

And where, for that matter, has the fitness movement left the estimated 80 to 90 percent of us who for one reason or another have simply watched the movement pass by? Could there be a low-level feeling of guilt associated with this spectatorship that is subconsciously stressful?

For all the stress the fitness movement has relieved, it's our guess that it has created a lot more. Between the missed workouts, the dreaded workouts, and the grueling workouts, it's doubtful that aerobic exercise has been the great psychological peace-maker that aerobic propaganda has wanted us to believe. Consider the case of Andy, for example:

"The regimentation is what kills it for me. Every time I try to get started with an exercise program, I feel like I'm being punished. The counting, the numbers. I'm only on my tenth push-up, knowing I've got twenty left, and a flash of depression comes over me that I just know is something I'm not going to be able to deal with on a regular basis. I don't understand how some people can get high from exercise. I get low from exercise. Maybe it's because I always wind up feeling guilty that whatever I've tried has felt so difficult. Exercise reminds me how much I've gotten out of shape."

Any of that sound familiar?

The Andy in this scenario is my brother, Andy Shimer. We played sports together all through high school, and Andy was one of the most naturally gifted athletes I've ever known. But after a few more glory days of football and wrestling in college, that was it. Exercise, without the rewards and the fun of a sport to go with it, was just too much of a stress for Andy to handle.

And me?

I took just the opposite route. I took the stress and ran with it—clocking a 3:15 marathon on my first try. Between the ages of twenty-eight and thirty-eight, I never missed, not even for a day, strenuous workout lasting at least forty minutes. Sick, injured, too busy—it didn't matter. I was owned and operated by an aerobic force.

Was it stressful?

It was crippling. My workouts were the biggest challenge of my day. Once they were over, everything else felt like clear sailing, whether it really should have or not. But heck, I was fit, and I had avoided the plight of my brother, Andy, who had put on thirty pounds in all the wrong places.

I was so "fit" that when I joined the Rodale Press as the editor of _The Executive Fitness Newsletter_ in 1978, I had a resting pulse of 34. The doctor recording the figure suspected some sort of coronary abnormality, so he ordered an EKG (electrocardiogram) and a stress test. I tried to explain that I had a pretty severe exercise habit that was probably responsible for my slow pulse, but he wouldn't have it. A week later I was sitting in running shorts on an examination table, sprouting more wires from my chest than hairs.

"The doctor will be with you shortly," a nurse leaned in to announce.

I knew that meant "kill some times," so I did. I started playing a little game with the monitor that was giving a digital readout of my heart rate. It was sensitive enough to jump a few points even if I just moved my arms, so I decided to see if I could get it to fluctuate by "moving" my mind. I thought about having a serious heart problem based on the test I was about to take and my pulse climbed 12 beats to 46. I imagined sitting on my back porch watching the sunset and it dropped back down to 35. I imagined the nurse in a bikini—40.

But what affected my heart rate far more than I would have expected was the mere thought of my daily workout. When I thought about how, even after running that treadmill, I'd be going home to run for forty minutes in a rubber sweat suit carrying 10-pound dumbbells, my heart rate jumped to 48. Could the stress that my workouts were causing me be hurting my health more than my exercise was helping it?

I didn't have the opportunity to dwell on this sobering thought, because the doctor arrived and I went on to display the "fittest" cardiovascular system he had ever tested in his ten years at the facility. The doctor's clean bill of health and enthusiasm for my extraordinary fitness relieved my mind.

But the issue resurfaced in 1987 when M. W. Buckalew, Ph.D., of the University of North Carolina at Asheville, revealed a provocative finding. Dr. Buckalew discovered that people who approached their exercise routines in a do-or-die, highly competitive fashion did not enjoy the same improvement in their cholesterol profiles as people who exercised in a way that was more relaxed and enjoyable. The HDL (good) cholesterol levels of the driven exercisers did not increase as much as the HDLs of the calmer exercisers.

Knowing that I fit Dr. Buckalew's description of a "do-or-die exerciser," I quickly got on the phone to Dr. Buckalew to get his thoughts.

"It's ironic that so many of us are killing ourselves to live longer when a less frenzied approach might better save the longevity goal," Dr. Buckalew told me. "It appears that a highly competitive attitude toward exercise may substantially limit the health benefits being sought."

It had been years since I had my cholesterol checked, so I had it tested to see if Dr. Buckalew's hypothesis applied to me. My HDLs were a lofty 71 mg./dl., almost 30 points above average. I dodged Dr. Buckalew's bullet, but the next one hit the bull's-eye. My total cholesterol came to 220 mg./dl. For a guy with 5 percent body fat and a 2:46 marathon to his credit, 220 seemed high. Add the fact that I had been avoiding red meat —and that my totally out-of-shape brother, Andy, had a cholesterol level of 150—and the figure of 220 seemed downright unfair.

Could the stress that my workouts were causing me in any way have been keeping my cholesterol elevated?

It's possible. Psychological stress can cause the body to release adrenaline, which in turn causes fat cells—especially those in the abdominal region—to release fat molecules into the bloodstream. This can put undue demands on the liver, whose job it is to process fat in the blood. The result: increases in the liver's output of cholesterol and LDL cholesterol, the bad kind especially. Research has shown that college students experience slight cholesterol increases during exam periods, and that accountants experience similar increases around the April tax rush. Could my stressful workouts have been doing the same to me? Could the constant feeling of dread I carried with me have been keeping my adrenaline levels high—and hence my cholesterol levels high—even though a good deal of that adrenaline was getting "burned off" by my workouts?

"It certainly makes sense intuitively," University of Virginia professor of psychiatry Robert Brown, M.D., Ph.D., remarked when I asked him for his opinion on the potentially negative effects of an overly burdensome workout schedule. He agreed that anxiety and dread can constitute a considerable stress, whether in the context of a bad relationship with a job, another person, or a monstrous exercise routine.

It's certainly something to think about for anyone whose exercise program is an especially onerous one. There may be a price to be paid for calling up the adrenaline it takes to get through a grueling workout, especially on a daily basis. Maybe it doesn't all get "burned off." And maybe just the dread of the workout keeps lesser levels of adrenaline flowing all the time.

Consider, too, the dangers of a dreaded workout not getting done. An emergency arises and suddenly the anticipatory adrenaline cannot be worked off. And what if this happens on a chronic basis? What if someone has made a commitment mentally to adhere to a strenuous exercise program but has difficulty following through physically? Does this person become a veritable adrenaline pond?

And could it all get even worse if the adrenaline from dread gets topped off with the stress hormones called into play by guilt?

It's new territory for exercise scientists, so no one is yet prepared to offer concrete answers. We do know, however, that personalities differ, and that the dread of a workout could manifest in ways quite different from a wave of adrenaline. Depression could set in.

But isn't exercise supposed to alleviate depression?

It can, but not when taken to extremes. According to Dr. William Morgan, of the University of Wisconsin, a pioneer in the field of sport psychology, ". . . healthy young men and women who are normal from a psychometric standpoint have, as a group, a significant increase in depression with heavy exercise. There is a dose/response relationship."

Too much of a good thing, in other words, can produce bad results.

The dread of the impending struggle can begin to defeat the purpose of that struggle. Physical activity can be an effective stress-reliever, but not if it constitutes a stress in its own right. Fighting fire with fire just doesn't work in the psychological world.

Do what you can to make your exercise enjoyable, or at least practical. Stop thinking there is anything inherently noble about the ability to endure pain. Pain needs purpose to be noble. Otherwise it's just plain stupid.

Expect specific advice on how to escape exercise addiction in Part IV.

8

Exercise for the Wrong Reasons

Stamford

Being entirely honest with oneself is a good exercise.
—Sigmund Freud, 1856–1939

Before we go any further, we should say again that we in no way mean to chide anyone for whom a regular exercise program has been working. If you honestly enjoy the solitude and feelings of accomplishment you get from jogging, or the camaraderie and flushed complexion you get from the exercise class or trips to the health club, or even just the privacy and chance for mind-wandering that come from pedaling a stationary bicycle or pulling on a rowing machine, congratulations. You're doing a good thing for your health and probably your happiness.

The problem is that there aren't a lot of people like you. Only a small fraction of the adult population exercises vigorously on a regular basis, and the number who enjoy their exercise is even less. I have met literally hundreds of regular exercisers in my work as an exercise physiologist at the University of Louisville and as a fitness instructor in the Louisville area, and while I can't say that all of these people despise their commitments, a good number of them do. I'm going to guess that only about 25 percent of the regular exercisers I've met fit into the category I call the "happies." These people are committed, but not compulsively so. They exercise to help preserve their health, but what keeps them going is the basic *pleasure* they derive from their exercise. They tend to go easy on themselves and are not competitive in what they do.

51

They also can miss a workout without experiencing any undue stress, which is an important characteristic. Happies seem to be well adjusted emotionally and also seem to be reasonably well satisfied in their professional lives.

After the happies come the "begrudgers." These people don't abhor the exercise they do, but they don't celebrate it, either. Usually they're exercising for a specific and legitimate reason—weight control or protection from heart disease, for example—but they're not compulsive about it and, like the "happies," they can miss a workout without feeling the world's going to end. My advice to these people is usually just to lighten up a bit. I suggest they add some variety, spontaneity, and fun to their workouts to lessen the load. I also recommend that they get involved in more activities that don't seem like exercise—the kinds of around-the-house chores, for example, that we'll be discussing in more detail later in this book.

Next, the "strivers." They exercise with a vengeance and not always lovingly, but I don't fault them for it because they usually have a specific athletic goal in mind. They are merely displaying the kind of dedication it takes to be a great collegiate, professional, or Olympic performer.

The regular exercisers I *do* find fault with, however, are the "compulsives." A compulsive is any exerciser who has lost control of his or her exercise commitment. That was me a few years ago, and I know from more than twenty years experience how devastating compulsive exercise can be. Compulsives exercise not because they want to or even because they feel they need to for health reasons. Compulsives allow a kind of superstition to build up around their workouts that robs the workouts of any logic. They simply must be done or unbearable psychological stress will result.

And worst of all is a subset of compulsives I call the "exorcisers"—those whose subservience to exercise is in effect a form of repentance for "sins" in the way they live. Exercise becomes an act of atonement for abuses that otherwise would cause the exerciser unbearable guilt. Sometimes the exorciser's feelings of guilt are deep-seated and reflect basic character disorders that may require therapy to roust out, but usually the guilt comes from shallower regions—too hefty a beer-drinking habit, smoking, an unchecked passion for chocolate chip cookies. Exorcisers want their vices and their good health, too, and they look to exercise as the ticket. Some examples:

"If I didn't drink, I don't think I'd jog at all. Jogging helps clear my head and I figure it burns off the calories."

—Bill, a forty-two-year-old car salesman

"I get some of my hardest workouts after my eating binges. I sometimes wonder if I'd be in the shape I'm in without them."

—Sue, a twenty-six-year-old beautician

"Sure I smoke, but I'm also the only golfer I know who carries his own clubs for the entire eighteen holes."

—Curt, a fifty-three-year-old real estate broker

Get the picture?

Maybe you get the picture all too well. And if you do, maybe you're taking sides with Bill, Sue, or Curt. What's so bad, after all, about a little misbehaving, especially if health-enhancing apologies are made?

If that's what were going on, nothing. But what Bill doesn't realize is that his jogging is doing very little to make peace with his liver, just as Sue's aerobics classes are not exempting her arteries from the saturated fat she engulfs when she binges. Curt lives the biggest lie of all. Exercise can do nothing to reverse the damage to the lungs or the arteries that smoking inflicts.

But at least these people are trying, you say. And besides, nobody's perfect.

I'm fully aware of that, because I'm certainly flawed myself. Our only point is that "exorcisers" should at least own up to the truth. Exercise is not the great eraser that many of us would like to think it is. At best, it's a modifier, and only because it can help keep weight down. It can do nothing to protect specific organs—the liver, heart, or lungs—from the specific attacks of alcohol, dietary fat, or cigarettes.

Worse yet, there's the perpetuation factor. If Sue believes her binges are actually helping her to be healthier by boosting her workouts, then her exercise isn't just stupid, it's an accomplice to a crime. The same goes for Curt and Bill. If they're using exercise to convince themselves their bad habits are not in fact bad, then their exercise is bad.

Matter of degree is important here, too, of course. There's nothing depraved about taking a slightly longer walk after dinner if the homemade pie demands a second helping. Trouble begins when you don't stop at the second helping and the walk becomes a 10-mile run. Especially dangerous is when the extra pieces of pie begin to feel justified by the 10-mile run. At that point you're into what psychologists call a closed feedback loop— a vicious cycle—which can be tough to escape.

We'll be talking more about exercise addiction in Part IV, but for the time being, how about a short quiz to see if exercise as a form of "exorcism" could be a problem for you? If you do nothing for exercise at all, feel free to skip the quiz. But if you are into a regular workout schedule, it certainly couldn't hurt to gain some insight as to why. We're hoping to help exercise addicts in this book, remember, not just exercise abstainers. Good luck with the quiz.

Do You Exercise or "Exorcise"?
Take This Test and Find Out

1. Is your exercise motivated by some sort of dietary indiscretion?
   (a) Rarely or never
   (b) Sometimes
   (c) Often

2. Is your exercise intended to counter the effects of drinking, smoking, or use of some illicit drug?
   (a) Rarely or never
   (b) Sometimes
   (c) Often

3. Does your exercise help alleviate feelings of anxiety or guilt that you can't quite seem to identify?
   (a) Rarely or never
   (b) Sometimes
   (c) Often

4. Do you exercise in order to feel you've accomplished something when in fact you're avoiding something you know you should be doing instead?
   (a) Rarely or never
   (b) Sometimes
   (c) Often

5. Do you feel you have to exercise before you can relax completely or feel worthy of enjoying such everyday pleasures as eating or interacting with other people?
   (a) Rarely or never
   (b) Sometimes
   (c) Often

6. If you cannot exercise for some perfectly understandable reason, do you feel a strong sense of loss anyway?
   (a) Rarely or never
   (b) Sometimes
   (c) Often

7. Does exercise help you overcome a gnawing sense of inferiority?
   (a) Rarely or never

(b) Sometimes
(c) Often

8. Do you enjoy your exercise while you are exercising?
   (a) Often
   (b) Sometimes
   (c) Rarely or never

9. Would you exercise in the same way you do now if there were no discernible outcomes such as improved fitness or a trimmer waist line?
   (a) Often
   (b) Sometimes
   (c) Rarely or never

10. Would you stop in the middle of your exercise routine to watch a sunset, smell the flowers, or chat with a neighbor?
    (a) Often
    (b) Sometimes
    (c) Rarely or never

Scoring: Give yourself a zero for every "a" answer, 1 for every "b" answer, and 2 for every "c".

- 0 to 5: Congratulations. Your reasons for exercising are probably sound and healthful.
- 6 to 10: Be careful. Your reasons for exercising could be held suspect.
- 11 to 15: A slap on the wrist. You may be doing more damage than good with your exercise.
- More than 15: Time for some serious self-examination. Your exercise has taken control of your life.

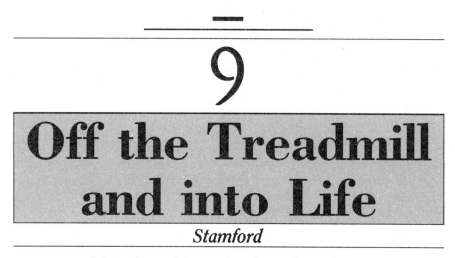

9

Off the Treadmill and into Life

Stamford

What a [person] has made, a [person] can change.
—Frederick Moore Vinson, 1890–1953

hile rigorous exercise certainly has its drawbacks, being totally sedentary also has its hazards. After all, exercise abstinence contributes far more than exercise abuse to the 725,000 deaths every year in the United States that continue to be caused by heart attack, stroke, and hypertension. Nearly 2,000 people die of cardiovascular diseases in this country every day. That comes to one person approximately every forty-three seconds. The numbers don't speak well for the heart-saving efforts of the fitness movement as they have been conducted so far.

So should we just preach the aerobic gospel with more zeal and more appeal? Make the aerobic shoe even softer and the leotards even brighter? Put more digital readouts on the rowing machines and run the Gut-Buster ad a few thousand more times on TV?

No doubt we will, but doubtful indeed is whether it'll make much difference. The fitness movement has been failing for some very fundamental reasons, and additional hype is not going to help. With all due respect to the fitness industry, overzealous marketing has been part of our fitness problem. We've been led to believe fitness can be bought when, of course, it can only be earned.

No, the solution to our fitness dilemma is not going to come from better fitness gadgetry, it's going to have to come from within. We're the

56

ones who created this hazardously sedentary lifestyle of ours; we're the ones who can change it.

But how? And why have we blundered so badly so far?

We've been looking to exercise as a Band-aid when our fitness problem has in fact been a tumor in need of major surgery. We've been grabbing for quick, aerobic fixes for something that for many of us has been a deep-seated problem not just of basic lifestyle, but of philosophy, priorities, and attitude. We want good health and the peace of mind it can bring, but we've not been willing to reach any farther than our toes to get it. The result has been the epidemic of heart disease, diabetes, hypertension, obesity, and stress-related illnesses that continue to plague us despite twenty years of aerobic first-aid.

I should know, remember, because I finally gave up on the aerobic "cure" myself despite having been a trusting patient for more than twenty years. A part of what finally did it for me, I think, was not just the sense of triviality in the time and effort I was spending, but the sense, too, of out-and-out contradiction. There I was, trying to preserve my life with my workouts when in effect my life was _passing me by_ because of my workouts. Maybe you've experienced a similar feeling if you've ever spent any time on a stationary bike or rowing machine that doesn't go anywhere. There you are, sacrificing precious moments from the present with the vague hope that it's going to pay off at some time in the future in the form of better health—or at least some thinner thighs. It's a tough way to stay motivated—and a downright counterproductive way if your life is passing you by in the process, as mine was. The best kind of motivation comes from the joy of doing, not from the obligation of doing and not from an expectation of some payoff in the future.

Blinded by the Sweat

I can assure you, however, that there was very little joy or usefulness in the workouts that used to control my life. Not only were they preventing me from seeing the "bigger picture" of where I was going with my life, they were blinding me to the smaller "snapshots" of which the bigger picture is made.

Not once on any of my runs, for example, do I remember focusing in on a beautiful aspect of nature. I had run at sunrise and sunset, and amid April showers as well as May flowers, but never once do I remember being uplifted by those experiences in the way that I can be uplifted by them now. The difference, you see, is that now I _walk_ parts of those old running routes, and I feel like Robert Frost himself when I do. Maybe I'm just not as smart as those people who can engage in deep thought at a seven-minute-per-mile clip, but I doubt it. I can tell you from Psychology 101 that pain and pensiveness are antagonists on a very basic level.

But before we all head out looking for jogging shoes to burn, let's realize that my compulsive approach to exercise was merely a reflection of my compulsive approach to life in general. I was—like many of us, I'm afraid—hell-bent for success, whether it was going to take me through fire and brimstone or not. I was totally captured by our nation's productivity ethic. "He who produces is valued—and the more the better—while he who produces nothing is worthless, expendable, a drain on society." I think it was the unconscious fear of not being valued that kept me going at a frantic pace. I was going to make a name for myself *and a name for exercise physiology* at the University of Louisville regardless of the price. I worked seven days a week, ten hours a day during my first years on campus—teaching a heavy load, doing research, writing grants and journal articles, coordinating community-based programs—and it paid off. I earned tenure in record time and became a full professor in eight years.

But was I happy?

In the beginning I thought so, and why not? I was being rewarded, respected, and praised. I had a successful career and a great physique. Why shouldn't I be happy?

The fact that I even started asking that question should have been my answer. I was highly successful yet highly dissatisfied. Regardless of what I would accomplish, it never seemed enough. I began even to be haunted by the suspicion that *because* I had succeeded at something, it must not have been all that difficult in the first place. No, I clearly was not happy even though that was not clear to me at the time. Only in retrospect can I see where I was going wrong. If I accomplished something it meant only that I had to tackle something even tougher the next time. I was on a treadmill to success that, like my treadmill to fitness, had only two gears—high and higher. And no "off" switch. No wonder I finally had to pull the plug.

A Lesson from the Less Privileged

I reveal all this not looking for sympathy, of course, but only with hopes that it might keep others from getting caught on a similar kind of conveyor belt. And my message applies to couch potatoes and exercise addicts alike. Many couch potatoes are couch potatoes, in fact, because they invest all available time and energy in the pursuit of vague plastic goals, leaving nothing for life itself, just as many exercise addicts pursue fitness to the point of leaving nothing for life itself. What we need is a better sense of balance. But no, we're a society that has been approaching personal fulfillment with the same "no pain, no gain" mentality that we've been approaching fitness, and with similar results. It's true that our standard of living has never been higher, but our rates of alcoholism, drug addiction, depression, suicide, and divorce have never been higher either. The parallel would suggest that we may need to give this thing we call success a second look. Are our goals really worth the price we're paying for them?

In my own case, my highly successful career was costly indeed. My first marriage finally failed after twelve stressful years, and my two sons grew to manhood while I was out jogging. I could have learned a great deal about life from them, but didn't. I have only a handful of good memories of years that could have been the most rewarding of my life had I been able to slow down enough to enjoy them.

My approach to life and my approach to exercise were the same. I could never work enough, write enough, run far enough or fast enough, or lift enough weight. More was better—always. Push, push, push. Just keep going and I would get there. But where was I going? I never stopped to ask.

Then I met (and later married) Joy Donaldson, and my life began to change for the better.

Joy is a professor of special education who has devoted her professional career to improving the lot of people who are labeled mentally retarded. By the time I came along, although she was still very professionally active, she had begun to choose her own professional activities on the basis of what she personally deemed worthwhile and valuable. She recognized that there is much more to life than a string of accomplishments. She sought balance and peace of mind. And she claimed that it was mentally retarded people themselves who had shaped her perspective on life. Through her I came to meet and to appreciate the very special qualities of these people—society's ultimate "dead wood"—who for the most part produce little and own nothing and yet are more open, honest, trusting, and optimistic about life than the rest of us can even hope to be. They know no competition, no malice, no symbols of status, and they could care less about looking like Sylvester Stallone or Cher, and yet they have a kindness, a nobility, and contentment that made me look at my own life in a whole new light. What was I so panicked about? Whom was I trying to impress? What goals did I have that were more important than the wonderful qualities these people had without so much as learning to read?

I'm not suggesting we all trash our ambitions or our IQ's, either—don't get me wrong. But I am suggesting that we examine our ambitions to see where they are really leading us and how they might be forcing us to feel more stressed than is necessary. A major aspect of our fitness failure has been that we feel so pressed for time. We want our fitness the way we want our food—fast—so we try to shrink exercise into short intense doses and cram it in where we can. The result has been the fitness fiasco that stares at us from our mirrors every day.

If we're going to get the kind of exercise that can work, that can be enjoyable and feel useful, that can relax us and bolster our feeling of purpose and self-worth, we're going to have to slow down enough to realize our priorities. Is the new luxury sedan really worth the overtime that's going to be running you ragged? Is the big house in the suburbs really worth the new job that's going to have you commuting an extra ninety minutes each weekday? Perhaps, in the thrill of the moment, the answer is yes. But soon, when the toll on your lifestyle cuts to the core, the answer will be a resounding NO!

The insights I have achieved from the variety of forces in my life can be distilled down to one thought: Life is a series of choices, and although we tend to feel powerless at times, a bare-bones look will reveal that at every turn we made a choice. We choose what to eat, where to go, and how to spend our money and time. What's more, we will continue making choices as long as we live. It's the little everyday choices that add up to a lifestyle. Realizing this truth at a deep level is powerful medicine for all that ails. Indeed, if you don't like the style of the life you're leading, you can change it. Perhaps not today or tomorrow, but gradually, with each little choice you make, you can change your life if you really want to.

John Schindler gives some advice in his best-selling book *How to Live 365 Days a Year* that goes a long way for a lot of us these days. It's the first and foremost of his twelve "important points to watch in living" and it states nothing more than "keep life simple."

It's a reverberation of Thoreau's classic observation: "That man is richest whose pleasures are cheapest"—wise words indeed for the times. Our waists have grown as large as the deficit in our national budget. It's time we trimmed down.

PHYSICAL ACTIVITY: FORGET THE SWEAT

10

Could You Be Fitter Than You Think? Take This Test and Find Out

Stamford

Sometimes the answer is right under your nose.
—Anonymous

en years ago, the idea of giving this test would have seemed like blasphemy to me. What kind of exercise physiologist—someone trained in the physiological blessings bestowed by strenuous aerobic exercise— would be suggesting that a Saturday morning spent cleaning out one's garage could do as much to protect against heart disease as a 3-mile jog?

And yet that's what the new research is suggesting. Findings from new studies demonstrate that modest physical activity affords similar protection from heart attack as vigorous aerobic exercise. The results of these landmark studies have not come as a great surprise because I have been seeing similar evidence day to day in my work at the University of Louisville. For the past fifteen years, I have been evaluating the health and fitness profiles of literally thousands of people, ranging in age from their teens to their eighties, and while I found it hard to accept at first that anyone could be healthy without getting enough exercise to be aerobically "fit," the evidence over the years simply became overwhelming. And I suppose I would have seen the writing on the wall even sooner had these people themselves not been under the impression that good health was impossible without strenuous exercise. They were coming to me, after all, for a health evaluation and exercise prescription because they believed health and fitness were one and the same. And, of course, my advice to these people had always been the party line: For the health that you're seeking, get your minimum requirement of at least three twenty-minute aerobic workouts a week or don't bother.

But those words, to be honest with you, now catch in my throat. After so many years of seeing nonexercisers come to me with healthy cholesterol levels, healthy blood pressures, healthy blood sugar levels, and healthy attitudes about life, I began wondering what I was supposed to fix!

The problem, of course, was that these people were simply too well informed. They were reading and believing the same aerobic doctrine that I was, so they believed they could only be half healthy if they weren't taking their aerobic medicine. And the real absurdity of it all was that by putting these people on strict exercise programs, most of which they failed at in short order, I was needlessly adding stress and guilt to their lives. I officially want to apologize for that. Relieving those people of their stress and guilt has been one of my major reasons for getting involved in this book. Yes, strenuous exercise has benefits, but it has no monopoly on those benefits. *Moderate* physical activity, a healthy diet, a healthy weight, and an optimistic, nonhostile approach to life can do all that an aerobic exercise program can do—and more. People who rely on exercise as an antidote for other glitches in their lifestyle are in for the rudest awakening of all. Strenuous exercise is a stress to the body in its own right. It's no way to counteract the stresses inflicted by a bad habit, a bad diet, or a hostile personality. But more on that in Part IV. Our purpose here is to find out if your current lifestyle is more "athletic" than you may think.

But before asking you to take a short quiz designed to put your own fitness levels into perspective, may I share with you two examples of the fitness-without-formal-exercise phenomenon. I can think of dozens, but these two stick in my mind most clearly. The first deals with my plumber, Mike, a large powerfully built man in his late thirties. The other is my own father.

First, Mike.

We had a problem with our drainage pipes several years ago that Mike informed me was "going to mean some digging." By "some digging" he meant a 4-foot by 8-foot hole at least 3 feet deep that would be needed to correct the situation. I shuddered to think what use of a back-hoe would cost, but that's not what Mike had in mind. He grabbed a couple of shovels off the truck and we went at it.

I had a lot of questions about what we were doing and why, but in all honesty I had to phrase them as succinctly as possible because I was finding myself running preciously short of oxygen. Mike's answers, on the other hand, were surprisingly elaborate. He was working as hard if not harder than I was, and yet he was describing my plumbing system to me with all the ease of a college professor at the podium.

"Do you work out?" I asked.

"How do you mean?" he said.

"Do you lift weights or jog?"

Mike went on to tell me that he used to consider himself in shape, but not since his high school football days, nearly twenty years ago. "I know I've really let myself go, haven't I?" he wanted to know.

All I could do was ask if we could wait until our lunch break to discuss it.

I shared this tale recently with Porter and he came back with a remarkably similar tale of his own. His plumber is Kermit, he's in his fifties, and he had humbled Porter more than once in similar ditch-digging competitions. "What is it with these guys?" we had to ask ourselves.

But of course we both knew darned well what it was with these guys. They were engaging in hard physical labor sometimes as often as five days a week. Portly though they were, they were in great shape. But neither considered himself to be an exerciser, and neither considered himself to be in good physical condition because neither could imagine himself running around the block much less running a 10 K or a marathon. It's an erroneous and unfair self-assessment made by more than just this country's plumbers, however. My years of fitness testing have taught me that more than a few hard-working housewives, carpenters, house painters, and avid gardeners have managed to keep themselves surprisingly fit. How my dad managed to keep in such good shape, however, continues to surprise me to this day.

My dad is many things, but above all he is a phenomenon of energy conservation. A tolerant man who never let much bother him, he gave new meaning to the word "stationary." He never pounded a nail, lifted a paint brush, sawed a board, washed a dish, or cut a blade of grass. When our mailbox once took a nose dive due to a rotted post, it was I, in the third grade, who finally had to prop it up with cinder blocks.

Dad was a machinist for Westinghouse, so no doubt he got some physical activity at work, but he sure didn't get any at home. Concerned about him as my education in exercise physiology began to progress, I would cajole him weekly to have a thorough physical. It was my plan to get him on a structured exercise program once he found out what a physical disaster he really was.

To shut me up more than anything else, I think, he finally gave in, though in retrospect I almost wish he hadn't. His blood pressure was great and he flew through the treadmill test like a spring chicken. "How'd I do?" were his only words when the test was over.

I have met and tested other people like my father since that day, and it's occurred to me that most have had three basic things in common: They've had a calm easygoing approach to life, they've been within 10 percent of their recommended body weight, and they have not been serious smokers. (Dad is a former light smoker.)

It's something to think about, certainly, as the media insists upon flooding us with new health advice every day. Genes fit into the picture, no doubt, as does the all-confounding element of chance, but if you look around you it's my guess you'll see a pattern in older people who've kept their good health: calm, trim, and smoke-free.

Could You Be Fitter Than You Think?
Take This Test

The purpose of this test is to find out if you are a fitness "sleeper," someone whose seemingly unathletic lifestyle is cutting the cardiovascular mustard better than current aerobic doctrine would suggest. If you do well on the test, congratulations, but don't rest on your laurels, because diet, "bad habits," and your outlook on life are perhaps even more important than how physically active you are. But more on that later.

And if you do poorly on the test?

Don't despair. In our next ten chapters we'll be showing how even members of the Couch Potato Hall of Fame can join the ranks of the fit —painlessly and even enjoyably. The key is in exercising the imagination along with the muscles.

And what if you're among the 10 to 15 percent of American adults who engage in formal aerobic exercise on a regular basis?

You're already as active as you need to be, but take the test anyway. You may find that you're getting enough physical activity in your day-to-day routine to make the workouts unnecessary.

Basic Activity/Fitness Test

1. In an average day, I climb ＿＿ flights of stairs (approximately twelve stairs per flight).

   (a) 1–5   1 point
   (b) 6–10   2 points
   (c) more than 10   4 points

2. My job requires that I be on my feet and moving ＿＿ hours a day (example: waitress, industrial inspector, nurse). Count actual time moving only—usually about half the time on the job.

   (a) 1 hour   2 points
   (b) 2 hours   3 points
   (c) 3 hours   4 points
   (d) 4 hours or more   6 points

3. My job requires that I be on my feet ＿＿ hours a day, but I move around very little (example: sales clerk).

   (a) less than 4 hours   0 points
   (b) 4 hours   1 point
   (c) 6 hours   2 points
   (d) 8 hours   3 points

4. In an average day I walk ＿＿ miles (walking at least 1 mile at a time without stopping).

   (a) 1 mile   2 points
   (b) 2 miles   4 points
   (c) 3 miles   6 points
   (d) 4 miles or more   10 points

5. I spend about ＿＿ hours a week tending a garden or lawn. (Points assume year-round activity. If seasonal, cut points in half.)

   (a) 1 hour   1 point
   (b) 2 hours   2 points
   (c) 3 hours   3 points
   (d) 4 hours   4 points
   (e) 5 hours or more   5 points

6. I am a parent who assumes primary responsibility for a preschool child. (Add 50 percent of points for each additional child.)

    (a) Child and parent at home all day   5 points
    (b) Child spends half day in day care center   3 points
    (c) Child spends full day in day care center   1 point

7. My job is physically demanding (lifting, carrying, shoveling, climbing) for _____ hour(s) a day. (Consider only the time you are actually involved in vigorous activity.)

    (a) 1 hour   3 points
    (b) 2 hours   5 points
    (c) 3 hours   7 points
    (d) 4 hours   9 points
    (e) 5 hours or more   12 points

8. I engage in light sports activities (doubles tennis, softball, volleyball) or dancing _____ hours a week. (Year-round activity is assumed, even though the sports may change. If the activity is seasonal, divide the points earned accordingly.)

    (a) 1 hour   1 point
    (b) 2 hours   2 points
    (c) 3 hours   3 points
    (d) 4 hours or more   5 points

9. I perform household chores (laundry, cleaning, cooking) an average of _____ hours a week.

    (a) 1 hour   1 point
    (b) 2 hours   2 points
    (c) 3 hours   3 points
    (d) 4 hours   4 points
    (e) 5 hours or more   6 points

10. I have a desk job, but leave my desk regularly to run errands, greet visitors, attend meetings, etc., at least _____ times an hour.

    (a) 6 times or less per hour   0 points
    (b) More than 6 times per hour   1 point

Scoring: Add up your total number of points.

- 11 or more points: Even though you are not engaged in a formal exercise program, chances are good that you are getting a sufficient

amount of physical activity each day. This is a plus, especially if you're covering your other health bases in terms of stress control, body weight, vice control, and diet.
- 5 to 10 points: You're probably in a little better shape than you think, but you can do much better.
- 0 to 4 points: You're a couch potato all-star and your health could be suffering for it. Try to build more activity into your life, no matter how trivial it may seem. The following ten chapters can help you.

11

Bringing Back the Brawn

Stamford

O! it is excellent
To have a giant's strength. . . .
—William Shakespeare, 1564–1616

When aerobic doctrine told us to hit the jogging trail to lose weight and prevent heart disease, it overlooked something very important: It overlooked muscular strength, and strength in the upper body especially. The message was that we could live by our legs alone, burning enough calories from the waist down to maintain weight control everywhere else. Just keep those legs moving, whether by jogging, cycling, or chasing a squash or tennis ball, and all else would fall into place.

But for millions it didn't happen. Arches fell instead. And knees went. And shins "splinted." And in women even some bladders, reproductive organs, and breasts suffered from the abuse. And for what?

The simple burning of the calorie. The concept of risking injury by doing the same activity over and over again merely for the purpose of burning calories seems a little absurd when you think about it. Why not burn calories in a way that's not only going to accomplish something, but will also help you be a better calorie-burning machine even as you're just reading the evening paper.

Impossible?

No. It just means using a little brawn. Aerobic exercise is great for burning calories, true, but it is not great for building muscle, which in many ways limits its weight-control value. Most of the calorie-burning

70

from aerobic exercise comes only as you do it. There may be a small "afterburn" effect if your workout has been a real killer, but the latest research indicates that the effect is probably negligible for most people. To wage war most effectively against fat, you need to be a good calorie-burning machine twenty-four hours a day, and having adequate muscle tissue is the only way to do that. Muscles are the chief energy burner in the body, whether they are working or not. At rest, muscles burn considerable energy just to maintain tone—a state of readiness. And when active, muscle can increase its metabolic rate by twenty-fold. Body fat, by comparison, contributes very little to energy expenditure. Muscle is clearly the best fat-fighting friend we have, but aerobic exercise does very little to encourage its growth.

But then how can marathon runners keep so fat-free? There's certainly not a lot of calorie-burning muscle on Bill Rodgers or Greta Weitz.

You wouldn't be asking that if you knew anything about what it takes to be a good marathon runner—usually two training runs a day totaling 12 to 15 miles. These people run for approximately 20 percent of their waking hours. And if they are forced to stop running due to injury, they tend to gain weight with alarming quickness if they do not cut back dramatically on their caloric intake. When you become exceptionally lean through a lot of aerobic exercise, you had better be prepared to make aerobic exercise a very big part of your life if you expect to stay lean. Take the case of Porter, for example.

When Porter was trying to make the football team during his freshman year at Princeton, he weighed a rock solid 175 pounds. As he found himself on the bench more often than in battle, however, he started skipping practices to go jogging. Pretty soon he was not only off the team, he was hooked, and by the time he graduated, he was down to 150 pounds.

Where had the weight gone, and in what form had it left?

The fact that Porter's maximum bench press had dropped from 240 to about 180 in those four years suggests that a considerable amount of the weight left in the form of muscle. Yes, he could breeze through the Boston Marathon in well under three hours, but he wasn't eager to be seen with his shirt off. Even his legs had lost muscle mass. Let's have a quick lesson in muscle physiology to see why.

There are two major types of muscle fibers—"fast-twitch" and "slow-twitch"—which lie side by side within each of the approximately 650 muscles in the body. When a muscle is exercised "aerobically," which means in a slow and rhythmic fashion that keeps it adequately supplied with oxygen, it is primarily the muscle's "slow-twitch" fibers that get called into action. These fibers gain in endurance from such activity, but they do not increase appreciably in strength or in size.

When a muscle is applied against considerable resistance, however, such as in lifting a ladder or pushing a loaded wheelbarrow, "fast-twitch" muscle fibers get the call, and these fibers *do* respond by increasing in size. This is why weight-lifters become so bulky. They are repeatedly subjecting their muscles to immense resistance and hence encouraging growth among their fast-twitch fibers.

So why had Porter's B.A. in jogging cost him 25 pounds of muscle?

By concentrating so heavily on aerobic jogging, Porter had allowed the fast-twitch fibers in his legs and arms alike to shrink through simple neglect. Had he supplemented his jogging even with some minimal resistance activity, he could have kept a lot more of his muscle mass than he did.

But who needs big muscles anyway, you say, especially if you're a woman? All you want is to be slim.

Careful. As I've mentioned, getting sleek by sacrificing fast-twitch muscle fibers to an overdose of aerobic exercise sets you up for trouble if you're not willing to make a lifetime commitment. Porter, as an example, finds he gains weight very easily now if he doesn't keep extremely active. He feels, in fact, that this is probably the biggest reason he's had such trouble curing himself of his aerobic addiction. By losing his muscle to aerobic exercise, he has become enslaved to that aerobic exercise as a weight-control strategy.

Currently we're working on getting Porter some of his old football muscle back with activities that require more of the strength that aerobic exercise does not, and it's working. He's been able to put about 5 pounds of muscle back on in the past year, and his house and yard are looking as much better as he is.

But if Porter's metabolism had become so enslaved to aerobic exercise, why hadn't mine? I, too, had been a addicted jogger, remember, but was able to quit "cold turkey" with no change in my weight whatsoever.

The answer to that only reinforces my point about muscle's fat-fighting effects. Even though I jogged, I continued to lift weights, off and on, at least one day a week during my aerobic imprisonment. As a result, I had enough muscle mass to protect me when I made my aerobic escape. I still lift weights one day a week, in fact.

If that sounds like a violation of our *Fitness Without Exercise* philosophy, it's not, because I enjoy the lifting and I do not go about it in the compulsive fashion that I used to. My two sons and I get together on Sunday afternoons in my garage, and it's a chance for enhancing our friendship as much as our fitness. I lift nowhere near the amount of weight I used to, and I don't count my number of repetitions. I just lift because it feels good. I never thought I'd be able to say that, coming from the "bust a gut or don't bother" school of athletic logic, but the time I spend lifting is now time that I deeply enjoy.

I also enjoy the results I'm getting. My own experience and research findings show that the body's fast-twitch fibers can retain their size and strength by being exercised just once a week. I'm not building any new muscle tissue with my once-a-week routine, but I'm doing a surprisingly good job of maintaining what I've already got.

But there's more than ego involved here. Studies show that the muscle mass of the average American decreases by 10 to 12 percent between the ages of thirty and sixty-five, and that strength decreases by about 20 percent. Beyond the age of sixty-five, this decline becomes an avalanche. Over one-quarter of American men and two-thirds of American women older than seventy-four cannot lift objects heavier than 10 pounds. Some of this loss is due to aging, but much of it is from pure neglect.

I intend to sustain a vigorous and active lifestyle well into old age, and I intend to continue eating all I want. In order to realize these goals, I make it a point to keep my fast-twitch fibers in shape.

But don't slow-twitch fibers also need attention to stay in shape?

Slow-twitch fibers get called upon by most minor tasks, which means that if you are the least bit active, you are using your slow-twitch fibers. This may be enough to sustain them well into old age. Not so with the fast-twitchers, however. Research shows that with age muscle loss is predominantly from the pool of fast-twitch fibers, and two kinds of loss occur. Each fast-twitch fiber atrophies (gets smaller), plus some fast-twitch fibers deteriorate completely. Atrophy can be reversed, and deterioration may be partially preventable, but only if the fast-twitch fibers are called into play at regular intervals. This takes effort beyond everyday movements.

The message is clear: Use those fast-twitch fibers or lose them, possibly forever.

All things considered, we might be a fitter nation right now if the aerobic movement had not allowed us to forget our fast-twitch friends. All we need to do is look back a few years. Our ancestors who settled this country remained lean and muscular without taking their lunch breaks to jog. They pushed, pulled, and lifted their way to fitness. It could be argued that our prehistoric ancestors achieved high levels of fitness in a similar fashion. It is unlikely, for example, that they frequently jogged long distances. Activities involving strength in the upper body were more likely to have made up the bulk of their daily endeavors.

RAs Are the Way

So what are we actually suggesting here?

Some loss of muscle and strength is inevitable with age—that's a fact of life. But when Jack LaLanne, to commemorate his sixty-fifth birthday, can tow sixty-five rowboats loaded with 65,000 pounds of wood pulp 1½ miles across Lake Osuoko in Japan—handcuffed—it's clear that a lot of us are letting Father Time take away considerably more of our strength than we need to.

Are we suggesting the kind of daily diet of push-ups that have been the key to Jack's miraculous durability?

Of course not. That would run counter to the principles of this book in addition to being a waste of time. What we do recommend, however, is something we're going to call "resistance activity (RA)." Not resistance training, but resistance *activity*—maneuvers that provide enough resistance to the muscles to keep them toned and strong, but not so much resistance that you puff and pant or subject yourself to undue risks of injury. You probably won't be building appreciable amounts of additional muscle tissue with these activities, but you will be preserving and toning existing fibers to a degree that should be able to boost your "round the clock" calorie-burning significantly.

And the activities that can do this?

Again, nothing elaborate, strenuous, or expensive. Many of the activities can save you money, in fact, because they're around-the-house chores such as raking, carpentry, splitting and stacking firewood, scrubbing floors, shoveling snow, moving furniture, and even just carrying grocery bags or kneading bread. Recreational RA's can include golf—if you carry your clubs—hiking in hilly terrain, gardening, water skiing, and downhill skiing. And let's not forget the workout gotten from attending the needs of a toddler. Lifting and carrying a baby will do every bit as much for your fast-twitch fibers as hoisting dumbbells.

And remember: Muscle mass and strength require relatively little attention to keep them going. Even by just throwing some 5- or 10-pound dumbbells around every few days, existing muscle mass can be preserved. The fast-twitch fibers are very amenable in this regard. They need only to be jostled periodically to be kept awake.

Consider, for example, the routine that my wife, Joy, does. No one hates to exercise more than Joy, so rest assured that her routine is not inconvenient, unpleasant, or a time waster. For the time it takes, in fact, a routine like Joy's may be one of the most efficient things you can do to preserve muscle mass and hence maintain a good fat-fighting metabolism. (*Caution*: Unlike activities such as walking, cycling, or light sporting activities, RA's should *not* be done immediately after eating, especially if the meal has been a large one. Wait at least two hours. Resistance activity tends to raise blood pressure in its own right, an effect that can be compounded by a full stomach.)

Joy's Two-Minute Muscle Saver

Joy uses a pair of 5-pound Heavy Hands in each of the following move-ments. You can go heavier or lighter as you prefer. You can also use household items such as plastic milk cartons filled or partially filled with water. Perform all movements slowly and under strict control. *Never* allow momentum to develop—it can injure the joint. Do as many movements as you like, but be sure to challenge the muscle somewhat before you quit. The entire routine requires only a few minutes.

- *Curls*—for the upper arms (biceps). Hold weights at arm's length at your sides, palms forward. Bend the arm at the elbow, keeping the elbow at your side. Raise the hand to your shoulder then return slowly to the starting position. You can lift both arms at the same time, or alternate movements left and right. Perform the same movement with the palms down to work the lower arms.
- *Presses*—for the upper rear arms (triceps) and shoulders. Hold the weights at shoulder height with palms facing your ears. Press weights overhead until elbows are straight, then return slowly to the starting position. You can press both weights at the same time, or alternate movements left and right.
- *Raises* (lateral)—for the shoulders and upper back. Hold weights at arm's length at your sides, palms facing your body. Bend the elbows slightly and raise both the arms to the sides. Stop when your arms are parallel with the floor. Lower slowly to the starting position.
- *Squats*—for the legs and lower back. Assume the starting position for raises. Bend at the knees until the thighs are parallel with the floor and return to the starting position. Before lowering again, and with knees straight, rise up on the toes ballerina style. Keep the arms straight throughout.

An Added Bone-us

Muscle mass and calorie-burning aside, research shows that bones and joints can benefit from resistance activity, too. Bone is living tissue that needs exercise to stay strong, just like muscle. Women especially need to keep this in mind because they undergo hormonal changes that promote loss of calcium. Research shows that women can begin to lose appreciable amounts of bone mass as early as age thirty-five, suffering losses of as much as 30 percent by old age. Bone loss in men generally starts at the age of about fifty, leading to losses of about 20 percent by old age. Aerobic exercise involving the legs can substantially retard these losses in the bones of the lower body, but to keep bones of the upper body strong, exercise involving the arms is needed, and that's where the pulling, pushing, and lifting characteristics of RA's can be of benefit. When muscles contract, they pull on the tendons, which connect muscles to bones, and the ligaments, which connect bone to bone. This in turn produces the stress that it takes to induce bones to produce new cells.

The same holds true for joints. Like muscles and bones, joints need stress to remain strong. Not too much stress, such as the kind jogging can produce, but certainly enough to keep them mobile. Mobility insures adequate flow of synovial fluid to the cartilage of the joints. As one rheumatologist describes the process, movement causes "intermittent compressions and releases by which synovial fluid enters and leaves the cartilage in very much the same way that air enters and leaves the lungs." An adequate flow of synovial fluid appears to be especially important for the prevention of osteoarthritis.

So stop thinking of your joints as things that wear out from too much use. If anything, they "seize up" with not enough use. The kinds of motions that resistance activities provide can protect joints by keeping them adequately lubricated with synovial fluid. Also, by keeping muscles strong around the joints, RA's can prevent the kind of stress overload that can lead to harm.

In conclusion, we'd like to say that muscular strength has probably been more important to human survival throughout the ages than aerobic endurance. The caveperson who could mount a successful self-defense, after all, didn't have to run. The ancient Greeks thought so highly of muscular strength that for a time they trained by lifting young bulls, growing in strength as the bulls grew. And to this day, it's sad but nonetheless true that being strong can be a deterrent to having sand kicked in your face.

Let's not forget those things as we pursue a fitness that can serve us in as many ways as possible. We live not by our legs alone.

12

How Much Activity Is Enough?: Target 2,000

Shimer

Enough: Sufficient to meet a need.
—The American Heritage Dictionary

If you're happy with your score on the fitness test in chapter 10 and you're also happy with the activities in your life that earned you that score, congratulations. With a good low-fat diet, a healthy attitude, and a reasonable approach to life's "vices," you may be doing as much as reasonably can be expected with the genetic hand you've been dealt.

But if you did poorly on the test, or if you did well but we've raised the concern that you may be overdoing it, we need to talk. Inactivity can be lethal, but sacrificing your life to a pair of jogging shoes has its drawbacks, too. The key to a long and rewarding life lies somewhere between the two—being fit enough to be healthy, but not being dominated by that fitness. Becoming the servant of an exercise program may build strength physically, but psychologically it can lead to weakness by becoming a crutch. You begin to lean on the rigors of the workout for your self-esteem rather than on the rigors of real life. Fitness should be a means toward an end rather than an end in itself.

Hence, the following chart. You'll see some standard forms of aerobic exercise here, but you'll also see lots of activities with potential for being constructive and just plain fun. *These, too, can count as exercise.* The key is to expend approximately 2,000 calories a week—an average of about 285 a day—in activities above and beyond your job. The 2,000-calorie figure, however, assumes that your job is essentially sedentary. If your job is quite physical, you may not have to worry about expending any additional calories at all. Such professions are not cakewalks, however. Only (non-loafing) construction workers, carpenters, plumbers, masons, electricians, house painters, farmers, lumberjacks, tree surgeons, landscapers, linesmen, movers, waiters and waitresses, and professional dancers and athletes earn exemption. That might sound like a lot of people, but it constitutes only a small segment of the total U.S. work force. The rest of us probably should *not* just put our feet up after work, even if it has seemed like a "hard" day.

But "hard" is not what our heart-saving activities have to be, either. Look over the following list. Choose what you like and ignore what you don't. Happiness should be your goal as much as health. Don't make the mistake of committing to something you're going to wind up resenting and then not doing. And don't be afraid of variety. It can be your key to consistency, and it also can be your key to getting to a greater number of muscle groups. Work in the garden one day for the shoulders and arms, and play a game of badminton or go for a walk after dinner the next day for the legs. Above all, however, *respect your needs for pleasure.* If the fitness movement has indeed gone belly-up, it's done so for failing to satisfy our basic RDA's for enjoyment. The idea of a tough workout after a tough day at work has simply been too tough for most of us to handle. Isn't it nice to know that *it's also unnecessary.*

Activities Dear to the Heart and Home

Our goal in putting together the following information has been to include something for everyone, both in terms of the variety of activities and the range in caloric costs of those activities. If math is not your strong point, simply assume that by averaging about thirty to sixty minutes a day of most of these activities, you will be meeting the RWA (Recommended Weekly Allowance) of 2,000 calories of leisure-time energy expenditure that the latest fitness research suggests is optimal in preventing heart disease. If you're one who likes numbers, however, and can be motivated by them, feel free to use our Body Weight × Calories Per Hour formula to determine your energy expenditures more accurately.

A word to the wise, however: Do not make the mistake of becoming as compulsive about burning calories around the house as some people have become about burning calories through aerobic exercise. That would defeat the most basic purpose of this book, which is to free you from regimentation. Be spontaneous. Think about what these activities can accomplish for the house and yard as well as for your health. Have fun! And do so with full assurance that by expending roughly 2,000 calories a week through these seemingly routine activities, you'll be doing as much good for your heart as someone who trains for marathons. That should certainly help get you away from the TV.

Using the Table

The values in the Target 2,000 table are presented for an average adult male weighing 180 pounds and an average adult female weighing 130 pounds. If you are not within 15 pounds of either weight, the values in the table will not be appropriate for you, and it will be necessary to do a few simple calculations that automatically correct all values for size—an important determinant of energy expenditure. (See the note on "How to Compute" on page 80.) Note, too, that the calories burned by any activity will vary according to the intensity of the effort applied to it. If you're a house on fire in everything you do, assume your values for these activities will be slightly higher. The values presented assume you are moving continuously at a comfortable pace.

To arrive at your weekly total, simply select the listed energy cost for each activity and the amount of time per week you devote to it. Go by any time increments that you feel most realistically and accurately apply—dividing the hourly figures by 4, for example, if fifteen-minute stints are more your style. Every little bit counts. Do not, however, give yourself the benefit of too many doubts, which can be a natural tendency. Dr. Charles Kuntzleman tells the story in his book *Activetics* of the nurse who estimated she walked 10 miles per shift. Outfitted with a pedometer, however, she proved to be legging only about 2. When in doubt, slightly downgrade your estimates.

We've included a few examples to help get you started. You're shooting, remember, for a total of 2,000 calories per week. That's optimal. But don't despair if you fall short. Research has shown that as few as 1,050 calories a week can decrease heart disease risk, and that some minimal health benefits can accrue even at lower levels. But if your activity level falls to 500 calories ("just about comatose," according to epidemiologist Dr. Ronald LaPorte), research shows you increase your risk of heart disease and premature death possibly by as much as by smoking a pack a day of cigarettes.

How to compute. Example: You weigh 150 pounds and you play badminton (energy cost of 2.6 calories per hour per pound of body weight) for two hours a week. Two hours × 2.6 × 150 lb. = 780 calories.

If you play only fifteen minutes per week, manipulate the numbers as indicated in the example below.

Activity	Hours/wk.		Cal./hr./lb.		Weight		Total
Badminton	2	×	2.6	×	150	=	780
Badminton	0.25	×	2.6	×	150	=	98

Target 2,000: Caloric Cost of Physical Activities

FUN ACTIVITIES	Hours/wk.	Cal./hr. 180-lb. male	Cal./hr. 130-lb. female	Cal./hr./lb.	Total
Badminton	————	468	338	2.6	————
Dancing (ballroom)	————	288	208	1.6	————
Dancing (disco)	————	468	338	2.6	————
Golf (walking)	————	411	299	2.3	————
Hiking (hilly)	————	648	468	3.6	————
Horseback riding (trot)	————	504	364	2.8	————
Racquetball	————	738	533	4.1	————
Scuba diving	————	684	494	3.8	————
Skating	————	468	338	2.6	————
Skiing (cross-country)	————	666	481	3.7	————
Skiing (downhill)	————	468	338	2.6	————
Snowshoe walking	————	810	585	4.5	————
Squash	————	774	559	4.3	————
Soccer	————	666	481	3.7	————
Table tennis	————	342	247	1.9	————
Tennis (singles)	————	522	377	2.9	————
Tennis (doubles)	————	324	234	1.8	————
Volleyball	————	396	286	2.2	————
Walking (2–2.5 mph)	————	288	208	1.6	————
Walking (3.5 mph)	————	432	312	2.4	————
Water skiing	————	540	390	3.0	————
DOMESTIC CHORES					
Carpentry	————	270	195	1.5	————
Carrying firewood	————	918	663	5.1	————

FUN ACTIVITIES	Hours/wk.	Cal./hr. 180-lb. male	Cal./hr. 130-lb. female	Cal./hr./lb.	Total
Chopping wood (ax)	_____	414	299	2.3	_____
Digging ditches	_____	701	507	3.9	_____
Farming (light)	_____	414	299	2.3	_____
Farming (heavy)	_____	576	416	3.2	_____
Gardening (dig, hoe)	_____	576	416	3.2	_____
Trimming hedges	_____	378	273	2.1	_____
Horse grooming	_____	630	455	3.5	_____
House cleaning	_____	288	208	1.6	_____
Mopping	_____	306	221	1.7	_____
Mowing lawn	_____	486	351	2.7	_____
Operating lathe	_____	252	182	1.4	_____
Painting (outside)	_____	378	273	2.1	_____
Paint scraping	_____	306	221	1.7	_____
Plastering	_____	378	273	2.1	_____
Raking	_____	270	195	1.5	_____
Sawing by hand	_____	594	429	3.3	_____
Sawing (power saw)	_____	360	260	2.0	_____
Scrubbing floors	_____	522	377	2.9	_____
Snow shoveling (light)	_____	702	507	3.9	_____
Stacking firewood	_____	450	325	2.5	_____
Stocking shelves	_____	270	195	1.5	_____
Trimming trees	_____	630	455	3.5	_____
Washing/polishing car	_____	270	195	1.5	_____
Weeding	_____	360	260	2.0	_____
Welding	_____	252	182	1.4	_____
Window cleaning	_____	288	208	1.6	_____
Stair climbing (per 12-stair flight)		4.5	3.3	.025	_____

EXERCISE

	Hours/wk.	Cal./hr. 180-lb. male	Cal./hr. 130-lb. female	Cal./hr./lb.	Total
Cycling (10 mph)	_____	486	351	2.7	_____
Jogging (6 mph)	_____	756	546	4.2	_____
Jumping rope	_____	684	494	3.8	_____
Rowing machine	_____	558	403	3.1	_____
Swimming (slow crawl)	_____	630	455	3.5	_____
Weight training	_____	342	247	1.9	_____

Grand total per week _____

Tag-Alongs to Aid Weight Loss

These activities, though mild, also can be health enhancers. They can add to the total number of calories burned in a day, and hence aid weight loss. If you've met your 2,000-calorie quota from the previous list, you might look to these lesser activities as adding bonus points, points that can be especially valuable if one of your goals is a slimmer physique.

Note: As a reference, consider that basal metabolic rate—the number of calories someone burns just sitting quietly—is about 75 to 80 calories an hour for someone weighing 150 pounds.

FUN ACTIVITIES	Hours/wk.	Cal./hr. 180-lb. male	Cal./hr. 130-lb. female	Cal./hr./lb.	Total
Archery	_____	234	169	1.3	_____
Billiards	_____	198	143	1.1	_____
Canoeing (2 mph)	_____	216	156	1.2	_____
Croquet	_____	234	169	1.3	_____
Fishing (standing)	_____	234	169	1.3	_____
Horseback walking	_____	198	143	1.1	_____
Playing accordion (sit)	_____	162	117	0.9	_____
Playing piano	_____	198	143	1.1	_____
Sex	_____	240	170	1.3	_____
DOMESTIC CHORES					
Baking	_____	180	130	1.0	_____
Carpet sweeping	_____	234	169	1.3	_____
Cooking	_____	216	156	1.2	_____
Food shopping	_____	234	169	1.3	_____
Ironing	_____	162	117	0.9	_____
Standing	_____	126	91	0.7	_____
Typing (electric)	_____	126	91	0.7	_____
Typing (manual)	_____	144	104	0.8	_____
Wallpapering	_____	234	169	1.3	_____

Grand total per week _____

Rethinking the Chore

But wait a minute. Maybe you can handle the idea of "playing" your way fit, but not the notion of becoming some sort of aerobic janitor. All you have to do is pick up a dictionary to know that a chore is "a difficult or disagreeable task." Where's the great news here? Maybe you'd *rather* jog or pedal a stationary bicycle than wallow in the unending indignities of household chores.

We hear you. We *are* you. My grass used to get so long that it would gobble up Barbie dolls as fast as my daughters could buy them. My attempts to arrest its growth would go little further than neglecting to rake the leaves in the fall.

But I've taught myself to look at chores in a more positive light. They are, in fact, good forms of exercise; some of them are great forms of exercise. Sure, they seem unending, but to be of any value aerobic exercise also has to be unending. With chores, at least you're doing something that's going to have to get done sometime anyway. It's tough to feel that same sense of immediacy about a stationary bike ride or a 4-mile jog.

If you deeply despise doing chores, ask yourself whether it's really the chore you hate so much or the frame of mind you bring to the chore—the annoyance of having to engage in yet another "waste of time."

Delete that phrase from your vocabulary. Chores are not a waste of time. Think of them as a "waste" of calories, but not of time. And you might try breaking chores up, as I now do, to make them seem even less onerous. I'll cut the grass for thirty minutes or so every day or two, rather than get grouchy in anticipation of a three-hour marathon. Maybe I feel better about the whole thing since I let go of my need for perfection. The job doesn't have to be perfect, because the stuff's going to be returning in a week anyway, I now tell myself—too short a time to warrant my heart and soul.

No, our chores haven't been the problem all these years; it's been our attitude about doing them. If we can lighten that, we can lighten the chores. They'll get done, because they have to, but they don't have to get us in the process.

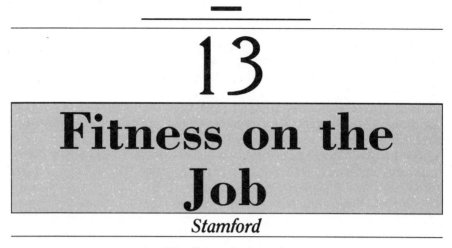

13

Fitness on the Job

Stamford

It's all in a day's work.
—Anonymous

Y our job. Whether you love it or loathe it, whether it feeds your ego or just your stomach, it takes a lot of your time. Eight hours a day is only the beginning if you're a professional or you own your own business— even if you're just trying to move up someone else's ladder. Add commuting time, "homework," and work-related social responsibilities, and it's easy to see why the fitness movement has had such a hard time fitting in. The idea of squeezing three aerobic workouts a week into the harried schedules of most white-collar Americans has seemed about as attractive as a hostile takeover.

But aren't office-bound Americans the ones buying all the rowing machines and turquoise running tights?

Buying is one thing, using is another. The fitness movement has made some blunders, as we've seen, but maybe its biggest has been to assume that people will work hard at fitness after already working hard at their jobs. Some will—and even like it and even begin to need it—but most will not. Unless the surveys are all wrong, most will come home, realize all the other things that have to be done, do them, and then feel deserving of at least some leisure time. Which is fully understandable. You can't argue with the priorities. You can, however, argue with how they're carried out.

We've talked already about being more physical around the house, forsaking some of the conveniences of technology for the more primal need of burning calories. That same strategy can be applied to the workplace. Whether you're a secretary or a vice-president, a factory worker or a traveling salesperson, you can fit more calorie-burning into your day. What's more, you can do it conveniently and in many cases even productively. The activities we recommend might not seem like much, but the advantage they can give you in your quest for weight control and/or a healthier heart can be immense over the long haul.

What many people tell me they like most of all about the "at work workout" philosophy is that it relieves them of the pressure they feel of having to burn all their calories at home. You're at your job for no fewer than eight hours five days a week, after all, and for the vast majority of that time you're doing nothing more physical than numbing your buttocks. Doesn't it make sense to use at least some of that time burning calories that you will then not have to burn at home? Even if you burn only 100 extra calories a day on the job, that's over a third of the way toward your daily goal of 285. And whether you do anything else for the rest of the day or not, it's still an extra 500 calories burned per week, enough to have you 7 pounds slimmer in a year—and all on "company time," which is what a lot of people find most attractive of all.

Could we be heading you toward a pink slip with the sort of job-site gymnastics we have in mind?

The answer to that ultimately will have to come from you, of course, but we sincerely doubt it. Considering that the activities we recommend can leave you feeling more energetic and alert, they may even help to further your career. Research has shown that a short walk, for example, is a significantly better energy-booster than a sugary snack. People in one experiment reported being noticeably more alert an hour after taking a brief walk than they did after eating a candy bar. Considering the calories as well as the energy difference there, the walk would certainly seem to be the more "career-wise" move to make.

So read through the rest of this chapter with an open mind. I must confess that I was once doubtful myself about the value of office exercise protocols, but necessity changed my thinking. Now office-bound myself, I seek out the corridors and stairwells at every opportunity. I supplement my work-site mobility with more activity at night and on weekends, but I'm convinced that the calorie-burning I manage to squeeze in between nine and five has been a major factor in my ability to keep my weight even a little lower than it was when I was taking time off in the afternoons to go for 5-mile runs.

A Word on Sweat: Get Warm but Not Wet

Before getting down to basics, however, we should probably address concerns you may be having about . . .

Sweat. Perspiration. Wetness. The stuff that's hard enough to control even without the added challenge of walking and stair-climbing. What's the boss going to think about the drip of perspiration that drops on his desk from the tip of your nose? And what are your cleaning bills going to be like for all those drenched dresses?

Relax. It's the thesis of this book that calorie-burning doesn't have to produce sweat, remember? I've been burning calories around the office for two years now, and I haven't stained a shirt yet. The trick is to keep efforts moderate and to keep them brief. What causes sweat is heat overload. The body sweats with hopes of being cooled by the sweat's evaporation. But without an excess of heat there's no need for cooling, so there's no sweat.

What causes nervous sweat, then?

Just that—nerves. Nervousness produces "apocrine" sweat, which is chemically quite different from the sweat (called "eccrine" sweat) produced by excessive body heat. Nervous sweat is chemically different enough from heat sweat, in fact, to attract bacteria in far greater numbers, as maybe you've noticed. Getting stopped by a police officer can leave you smelling a lot worse for wear than playing a set of tennis.

The office antics we have in mind have very little potential for producing either type of wetness, however, and may even help to minimize the nervous type by helping to dissipate stress. So here's the game plan if you're interested.

Calorie-Burning in the Corridors

Before you so much as tighten a shoelace, keep two things in mind: *Don't be too ambitious*, and *think long-term*. What you're trying to do is establish a habit, and just as habits are hard to break, they can be hard to start. So be patient with yourself, but don't be a push-over, either. If you can incorporate even just one of the following activities into your office routine within a period of about a month, consider that you've done well.

☐ *The mini-walk.* I've mentioned it before but I'm mentioning it again because it can be a miracle-worker. It also may be your best bet for initial success, and it won't attract attention—walking in the hall or up a flight of stairs is as natural as it can be. Just appear to be "going" somewhere.

The hardest part of mini-walks is simply remembering to do them. I suggest you come up with a system to cue yourself. A watch with an alarm can work, or you can try a desktop hourglass, or you can use your secretary if you've got one.
Frequency?
It's totally up to you.
Length?
Again, you're the boss. I've gotten accustomed to perhaps eight to twelve mini-walks a day, each lasting but a few minutes, but don't feel obligated to match my schedule. Remember that anything you do in the beginning is going to be better than nothing, and that your job, after all, does come first. Go for mini-walks only when time permits, and if you can fit a flight of stairs or two into a mini-walk, better yet. On nice days you might even want to treat yourself to some fresh air, especially if you're under stress. I've found the mini-walk can be amazingly therapeutic in this regard. Breathe deeply as you walk; let your arms swing freely, and smile, if at all possible. It's hard to stay hostile when you're smiling. Research suggests that activating the smile muscles also may stimulate chemicals that bolster the immune system, so consider the possibility of returning "re-inforced" in more ways than one after a mini-walk.

□ *Use the mini-walk to exercise creativity.* Besides calorie-burning and stress relief, mini-walks also can help creativity kick up its heels. Some of our greatest thinkers were avid walkers—Plato, Thomas Jefferson, Albert Einstein, Ralph Waldo Emerson, Charles Dickens, Bertrand Russell —and there's evidence to suggest that something more than fresh air may have been a factor. Some research argues that walking with a natural arm swing can aid communication between the left and right sides of the brain, which can pay big dividends in the blossoming of new ideas. Because the left side of the brain deals primarily with rational linear thinking, and the right side handles our intuitive, metaphorical ramblings, it can be a great idea to get the two together with help from the rhythms of walking. It sure seems to work for me. I get some of my best ideas when I'm walking freely, simply letting my mind wander. It's worth giving a try the next time you're sitting at your desk wrestling with a problem that seems hopeless. It might simply need help from both sides of your noggin.

But are mini-walks for "bigwigs" only, bosses who can come and go as they please?

They're easier for VIPs, certainly, or for those who govern their own work schedule, but they are still possible for those of us who need to "man our posts." The solution is simply to take "long cuts" to the restroom and to do less talking and more walking on coffee breaks.

□ *Do more standing.* It might seem insignificant, but the 10- to 20-calorie-an-hour difference between standing and sitting can add up. By standing instead of sitting for an hour a day, you could burn an extra 3,650 calories a year—enough for a fat loss of slightly more than 1 pound. By engaging in some stretching as you stand, you can burn even more calories and help dissipate stiffness as well. Reach for the sky, bend forward slowly, bend from side to side, bend backward. Do some imitation "backstroking." Bend at the knees slightly and hold for a few seconds. It might not seem like much, but it will get considerable amounts of blood moving through areas that will much appreciate the favor.

☐ *Pace when appropriate.* Just as standing burns more calories than sitting, pacing burns more calories than standing—about 1 calorie for every fifteen steps taken. You can pace when on the phone or pace when contemplating the solution to a problem.

☐ *Fit more stair-climbing into your day.* As we've seen elsewhere in this book, stair-climbing is as stellar an exercise as any. Figure on about 4 calories burned for every ten to twelve steps climbed—more per hour than hard jogging. If you have elevators in your building, either avoid them or ride them only part way to your destination. Very motivational, indeed, can be the calculation quoted earlier, by two doctors from Johns Hopkins, that the cardiovascular benefits of stair-climbing may amount to as much as four seconds of extra life for every step taken!

☐ *Communicate face-to-face.* Why tie up the phones to contact someone in your building when a visit in person can burn calories as well as "build some bridges" by making a better impression?

☐ *Park far from the "maddening" crowd.* Not only is your car less apt to suffer a mishap, you can burn as many as 20 to 30 extra calories a day by hoofing it to and from a remote area of your company's parking lot, or from a street a block or two away from your business.

☐ *Seek paths of greatest resistance by doing office isometrics.* I used to scoff at the old "door jamb press," but it can work, as can doing "curls" for the biceps by pulling up from beneath the lip of your desk. Exertions of just six seconds each, repeated five or ten times, aren't going to have you putting any beach bullies in their place, but they will help to keep muscles toned.

The Blue-Collar Advantage: Use It, Don't Abuse It

And what if your collar is blue—and frequently sweat-soaked, no less? Could you be getting enough activity on the job to exempt you from having to do much more than take your shoes off when you get home?

Very possibly. Both Porter and I have paid enough blue-collar dues to be able to vouch for the rigors of blue-collar labor personally as well as scientifically. One summer spent working in a car wash—in the days before automation; others spent moving furniture, bussing tables, or stocking shelves, plus janitorial work and washing dishes after classes taught me all I need to know about the demands of those lines of work. And Porter's experiences as a stone mason, house painter, and tree surgeon taught him respect for those trades.

Blue-collar America needs to beware, however, because the benefits of work-site exercise can be erased quickly at the dinner table and/or bar. Research shows that despite greater activity levels on the job, blue-collar workers suffer more from heart attacks, strokes, and high blood pressure than their more sedentary white-collar counterparts. Shoddy health habits off the job appear to be the reason.

Keep in mind, too, that not all blue-collar jobs are muscle-building monsters. The disappearance of exercise from the American workplace, after all, is what got the aerobics movement off and running in the first place. Less than a century ago, fully one-third of the energy responsible for powering the U.S. economy came from human muscle, but today that figure has dwindled to about 1 percent. Automation has turned a lot of broad shoulders into bay windows out on the farm just as it has converted a lot of iron-fisted factory workers into creampuffs. Be honest enough to admit if technology has taken the sweat out of your job. If you are not on your feet for the better part of your eight hours—and at least moving, if not necessarily bending, lifting, or carrying—you probably are not getting enough activity on the job. Some after-hours puttering around the house and yard may be as advisable for you as the guy with the potbelly who makes out the payroll. Consult the chart that concludes this chapter if you're in doubt about just how much activity your profession provides.

So what's our message to blue-collar America?

Simply this: Do not turn a potential advantage into a disadvantage. The benefits of even the most demanding job can get erased in the mere seconds it takes to engulf a jumbo cheeseburger or grab a smoke. Live healthfully, however, and your blue-collar job can be of great service to you. How many white-collar joggers can say they're being paid to exercise?

Better yet, by subscribing to the dietary advice of this book, and possibly even picking up on some of the at-home activity tips we give, you stand to widen your health advantage over white-collar America even more. Your steel-toed workshoes give you the chance to enjoy the best of both worlds. Don't blow it with an after-hours lifestyle that could stop Paul Bunyan, not to mention Archie Bunker.

The Calories Blue-Collar Work Can Burn

Could your job be keeping you fit?

This chart can help you find out. If your job burns more than about 150 calories an hour, you may not need to supplement it with more calorie-burning activities at home. Notice we say "may," however. A job that covers the activity component of the good health formula does nothing to satisfy the all-important elements of diet and vice control. If you have a voracious appetite, your on-the-job exercise may not be enough. And no exercise is enough to offset the hazards of smoking or alcohol abuse. Then, too, there's the issue of your physique. Even though you may be burning enough calories on the job to satisfy your heart, you may not be burning enough to satisfy the way you would like to look. If that's true, you may need to supplement your activities on the job with the kind of "exercise" opportunities we recommend in this book. If not that, you're going to have to eat less, or possibly come up with a combination of the two. (As a reference point for the following figures, consider that a 150-pound person burns approximately 75 to 80 calories an hour just by sitting.)

Calories burned per hour by someone weighing 150 pounds.
(Figures will be slightly higher or lower for someone weighing more or less.)

LIGHT WORK

Less than 150 calories per hour (average 140)

Bartending, slow
Checkout clerk
Washing dishes by hand
Driving a truck, light
Working with light hand tools

MODERATE WORK

Greater than 150 but less than 250 calories per hour
(average 220 calories per hour)

Assembly-line work, light
Bartending, busy
Bricklaying
Waiter/Waitress
Chain saw work
Carpentry, light
Domestic work—cleaning windows,
mopping, scrubbing floors
Driving a truck, heavy—including
getting on and off frequently
Electrical work
Farming—using modern equipment
Gas station attendant
Car mechanic
Masonry—plastering walls
House painting

Paperhanging
Stocking shelves
Washing and polishing cars
Welding, light
Window washer

HEAVY WORK

Greater than 250 calories per hour (average 375)

Assembly-line work, heavy
Carpentry, heavy
Pick and shovel work
Jackhammer work
Stacking lumber
Stone masonry

14

Fitness Around the House

Shimer

The house of every one is . . . castle and fortress.
—Sir Edward Coke, 1552–1634

What's got four walls, a roof, a yard, and the potential for offering more forms of exercise than any fitness device ever designed?

Yes, the average American home. Between the sweeping, dusting, scrubbing, scraping, painting, polishing, shoveling, raking, pruning, sawing, hammering, watering, and weeding, there's not a muscle of the body that could go untouched.

Yet where have millions of American homeowners felt they've needed to go for their workouts?

To the roads for a jog, or to a health club, or to a rowing machine, stationary bicycle, or exercise video. The aerobics movement has created a veritable exodus away from the household chore as a form of exercise. We'll hire Bob's Lawn 'n Leaf Service so we can get a "real" workout at the helm of something with chrome handles.

And why?

For some of us the lure of an "athletic" environment has been a factor, but if you examine the issue more closely, you'll find the concept of the "target heart rate" popping up. We've been told that building protection from heart disease depends on sustaining a heart rate of at least 60 percent of maximum for a period of at least twenty minutes, three times a week. Anything less goes for naught.

So where did that message leave this country's millions of home-owners who had grass to cut, shutters to paint, and hedges to prune?

It left them thinking that undertaking household chores put their homes ahead of their hearts. Sure, these activities produced a nice feeling of fatigue at the end of a day, but homeowners across the land knew they were fooling themselves to think that their aerobic requirement was being met. Bob's Lawn 'n Leaf, health clubs, and jogging shoe sales all began to flourish at once.

To which we say, "Come back home, America! Your lawn, your leaves, and your soiled floors can save you. Calories burned around the house can count every bit as much as those burned at the gym."

We've got to start looking at our homes less as fitness enemies than as fitness allies. They present us with countless opportunities for exercise that we tend to view only as annoyances. Whether it's a clogged toilet, a hole in the roof, shutters that need paint, or a rain gutter backed up—hey, it's exercise, a calorie-burner, a step toward a healthier heart. The latest research, as you'll recall, has found that as little as thirty to sixty minutes a day of light to moderate activity around the house and yard can reduce risks of fatal heart disease as much as an exercise routine that adheres to the aerobic rules. It's something to keep in mind the next time you're tempted to take your car to the automatic car wash.

Which brings us to perhaps the best reason of all to be active around the house—the cents it makes. Make a list sometime of all the routine maintenance and cleaning chores you tend to pay other people to do simply because you'd rather not be bothered with doing them yourself. Add to this the cost of any major renovation projects you may have contracted out over the years instead of tackling yourself. The total, if you're like most people, will leave you somewhere between shocked and ashamed.

Your home, if you own it, is the single greatest source of equity you have, so what could make more sense than to get it in shape as you get yourself in shape? We hereby nominate the American home as "exercise device of the year" for having the unique ability to bestow rewards finan-cially as well as physically for working on it.

Are You Hiring Your Heart Away?

The following are rough estimates of calories (and dollars) burned per hour on various household chores. Many services that we pay others to do could pay us as very worthwhile forms of exercise if we'd only start doing them. Remember, research shows that a caloric output of 2,000 calories a week (Target 2,000) invested in leisure-time physical activities can significantly re-duce risks of heart disease. So view these activities with that in mind. Figures given are for someone weighing 150 pounds. Consult the Target 2,000 table in chapter 12 for additional household activities not covered in this list.

Activity	Calories burned per hour	Dollars per hour to have done professionally
Bricklaying	205	15–25+
Carpentry	225	15–25+
Chain saw work	220	10–20
House cleaning—mopping, scrubbing, and washing windows	150–250	5–10
Electrical work—rewiring	240	15–25+
Lawn mowing—with push-type rotary	300–400	5–10
Making beds	135	5–10
House painting (inside)	135	10–15+
House painting (outside)	315	10–15+
Paperhanging	190	15–30
Raking leaves	225	5–10
Wood chopping (ax)	345	5–10
Gardening—weeding, hoeing, digging, spading	300–450	5–10
Pick and shovel work	585	10–20

The 10-Pound, 10-Week, Money-Saving "Deck Diet"

A true story: Ned wanted to lose 10 pounds one summer, and he also wanted a state-of-the-art deck built around his above-ground pool. He wanted to save money, too, so he came up with the following plan:

Ned would hire a contractor to do the job if the contractor would let Ned work along at a savings to Ned of $10 an hour. Ned convinced the contractor that he was quite handy, so the contractor agreed.

Ned determined that if he worked hard, he could burn 300 calories an hour, approximately 200 calories more per hour than he would burn by sunbathing or watching TV. For the ten weekends the contractor calculated it would take to do the job, Ned calculated this would come to 32,000 calories—1,600 for each of the eight-hour Saturdays and Sundays he would work. Because a pound of fat requires 3,500 calories of effort to burn off, Ned calculated that the ten weekends projected would account for a weight loss of about 9 pounds, maybe an even 10 if he worked some overtime.

Given the $1,600 Ned would be saving in the deal, he was very excited about the project.

Did it work?

Almost. Ned lost 8 pounds, and could have lost more if he and the contractor hadn't capped off each workday with several beers.

But a job well done nonetheless.

Does Ned's "Deck Diet" give you any weight-loss-through-work ideas of your own? You don't have to go to the extent Ned did to cash in on the concept. Even just a small garden can add valuable exercise in addition to some great low-fat nutrition. Or how about vowing to give your clothes dryer (and electric bill) a summer vacation—or the kid who cuts your grass?

The Calories Courtesy Can Burn

We miss out on burning calories around the house by avoiding more than just chores, however. Often we miss out through simple day-to-day laziness or lack of consideration for the other people with whom we live. For example:

- Neglecting to help bring groceries in from the car. Depending on the size of the shopping trip and carrying distance involved, figure on between 15 and 30 calories being involved—enough for a weight gain of about a pound if avoided three times a week for a year.
- Failing to help with cleanup in the kitchen. Figure on losing out on about 40 calories here if cleanup were to take about fifteen minutes. This misdemeanor, once a day, could penalize you with a weight gain of about 4 pounds a year.
- Shouting from a sitting position rather than getting up and going to another room to state one's case in person. Depending on the size of the person shouting, as many as 3 calories could be kept rather than burned here, enough for a weight gain of more than a pound of fat if done five times a day over the course of a year.

Get the message? The expression "It's the little things that count" makes sense in terms of calories as well as courtesy. Lack of consideration can add up in more ways than one.

15

Fitness Through Sports

Stamford

For when the One Great Scorer comes
To write against your name,
He marks—not that you won or lost—
But how you played the game.
                    —Grantland Rice, 1880–1954

The jogger passes the softball game with a snicker.

The swimmer stops to check his pulse.

The cyclist in knee-length shorts rides with a grimace rather than a grin.

What's going on here? What happened to the fun? What gave the fitness movement the right to ask us to keep an eye on our heart rates when we were just learning to keep our eye on the ball?

Good questions. "No pain, no gain" pinned a death sentence on fun sports, which may never earn parole. Better to go for a hateful 3-mile jog and then sit down to the stereo than to waste two hours on the softball field.

But is it? Let's do an instant replay and look at the facts:

Two hours of softball, providing they're not also spent drinking beer and eating hot dogs, burn about 500 calories for someone weighing 150 pounds. Pitchers and catchers can burn more—about 780 calories in two hours. A 3-mile jog, by comparison, followed by ninety minutes of relaxation burns only about 420 calories. The softball wins.

But the softball isn't "aerobic," you say?

As we've pointed out previously in this book, and as we will continue to point out for as long as it takes to get the point across to an aerobically biased America, motion is what burns calories, not misery. You could stick yourself with a pin and it wouldn't burn any calories. It might let a few out, but it wouldn't burn any. The kinds of activities that research has found to be so encouragingly protective against heart disease have not been aerobic, which means they have not been of sufficient intensity or continuous enough in nature to sustain the required "target heart rate" demanded by aerobic doctrine. And yet the activities are burning calories and exercising the muscles and giving healthy stress to the bones in ways that are adding up to substantially reduced rates not just of heart disease, but of premature mortality across the board.

Motion, not misery. It's a good phrase to keep in mind in light of the whip-and-chain athletic upbringing so many of us have had. When the going gets tough, the tough may get going, but the smart find an easier way.

Forget My Pulse, Give Me the Ball

I've seen the phenomenon countless times in my career as both an exercise physiologist and fitness instructor. Some people who can't even stick to a walking program jump out of their easy chairs like thoroughbreds when enticed by the challenge and the fun of athletic competition. Consider the case of Carol, an overweight woman in her early thirties who had been a casualty of one of my structured exercise classes back in the seventies. I saw Carol at a picnic several months after she had dropped out of my program and there she was, all 170 pounds of her, leaping and lunging in a volleyball game as I had never thought possible. Red-faced and sweating, she probably burned more calories in that hour than in any other hour of her adult life.

This isn't to say that heart-healthy sports have to beat you up, however. Any activity that gets you off the couch and away from the corn chips is going to be of significant cardiovascular value. As an example, in my work with the Kentucky State Troopers, mentioned earlier, a surprising number of these men demonstrate fitness levels well above what could be expected for the amount of physical activity they get on the job—recreational sporting activities being one of the biggest reasons. Some of the troopers are active gardeners and wood-cutters in their off hours, but I also hear talk of softball, hunting, basketball, and golf.

The point is that many of these men and women spend their leisure hours actively rather than passively, and it shows. Despite jobs that are for the most part sedentary, many display relatively low levels of body fat, healthy blood pressure, and healthy cholesterol levels. They're getting their fitness through fun.

As you can, too. If you're a person with sporting blood, use it. And use it with the confidence that you're doing your health a considerable favor whether you're sustaining a target heart rate or not. You're burning calories. And you're not into the vanilla fudge ice cream.

Fitness Through Fun

The following sporting activities can make a valuable contribution in helping you to meet your 2,000-calorie RWA (Recommended Weekly Allowance) of physical activity in your leisure time. Values are for a 150-pound person.

Activity	Calories burned per hour
Softball	250
Archery	195
Golf—walk, carry bag	345
Bowling	175
Tennis (singles)	435
Tennis (doubles)	270
Badminton	390
Horseshoes	180
Croquet	195
Ping Pong	285
Hunting	250
Fishing	195
Touch football	420
Canoeing	180

16

Fitness with the Kids

Shimer

Backward, turn backward, O time, in your flight,
Make me a child again, just for to-night!
—Elizabeth Akers Allen, 1832–1911

It's 10:00 A.M. on a typical Saturday morning in the upscale Arnold house. Mrs. Arnold, thirty-seven, is engrossed in sustaining a heart rate of 130 for thirty minutes on her new computerized exercise bike. Mr. Arnold, forty, is off on a 12-mile training run with a friend in preparation for an upcoming marathon.

Where are the kids?

They're snacking on Cocoa Puffs in front of the TV, watching "Pee Wee's Playhouse." James is nine and Christy is seven, and they've been watching TV since 8:00. After "Pee Wee's Playhouse," it will be "Garfield and Friends," followed by "Bugs Bunny and Tweety," followed by "Teen Wolf," followed by lunch.

Lunch will be hot dogs, potato chips, and chocolate milk (a meal that comes to 64 percent fat), followed by a trip to the video store for a movie, maybe two, to occupy James and Christy until dinner. Mr. and Mrs. Arnold will have broiled fish, baked potatoes, and steamed broccoli, because they're watching their weight and cholesterol, but James and Christy will have grilled cheese sandwiches and french fries (66 percent fat) and chocolate sundaes (62 percent fat) for "getting along so well" all day.

Which leaves what for Saturday night?

An evening out with friends for Mr. and Mrs. and a baby-sitter, more

99

TV, and plenty of buttered popcorn (52 percent fat the way the baby-sitter likes it) washed down by cream soda for James and Christy.

And so goes another Saturday not atypical of millions of American children. No wonder two-thirds of all kids between the ages of six and seventeen are "unfit" according to fitness experts. Or worse yet, that 40 percent of our children display a major risk factor for heart disease (high blood pressure, elevated cholesterol, or a weight problem) by the age of eight. Whatever fitness efforts we may be imposing on ourselves, we're doing a very poor job of sharing with our children. Is it because we think our kids are somehow immune that a diet of Pop Tarts, Sloppy Joes, and Three Musketeers gets turned into health food by some magic act of youth? Or that twenty-five hours a week of television (the national average) somehow gets compensated for by an hour a week of standing around in gym class?

At the rate things are going, the future does not look bright for the fitness of our children. Studies show that if a child remains obese through adolescence, the odds are three out of four that he or she will go on to be an obese adult. Couple that statistic with the fact that adolescent obesity currently is at an all-time high, and you can see why there's cause for concern.

Especially disconcerting is that we, as parents, appear to be failing our children from two directions. Research shows that we exert a negative influence if we are grossly unfit, but that we also do a disservice if, like the Arnolds, we pursue fitness to the point of subjecting our children to neglect. The classic question arises: What's a parent to do?

Being parents ourselves—Dr. Stamford has two sons and I have two daughters—we felt some personal opinion would not be out of line here. It seems to us that what may appear to be a dilemma is actually a great opportunity. If the kids need more physical activity—and you do, too— why not join forces? Or if the kids are vegetating while you're exercising yourself ever deeper into a fitness rut, why not use the kids for some variety? My two daughters are helping me do that right now, in fact, as part of my own rehabilitation from "fitness-itis." Just yesterday I cut my workout short to go skate-boarding with my seven-year-old. And this weekend I'll be going cycling with my twelve-year-old.

I've also got projects around the house planned for this summer—a tree house, a swing set, a brick patio, and, of course, our garden. The calories these things burn are very real, and the interaction with the kids gives a much better and longer-lasting "high" than any endorphins can. It can be a little trying sometimes—I'm not going to lie about that—but that's all part of the challenge. I can remember my seven-year-old last summer wanting to help paint the garage. It was important not to be sloppy because we were working precariously close to the prized flower bed of a fussy neighbor, so I let Sarah handle the "important" job of priming the garage with water. We were using latex paint, so it did serve a purpose other than just giving her some fun . . . and some good exercise.

If you use your imagination and are willing to display some patience, kids really can be great fitness companions. You may find one thing out pretty quickly, however, and it can be humiliating if you run into it the way I did. Kids have an amazing capability for cardiovascular endurance. It's explainable by the largeness of their hearts and lungs in relation to their often spindly little arms and legs, but I can tell you that spindly little arms and legs were all I could think about for weeks after entering a mile race with some "junior" track stars a few years back. It was during the early phases of my marathoning career, a track meet under the lights one summer night at the local high school. I entered in the "open" category, not knowing that "open" applied to a group of inner-city nine- and ten-year-olds as well as to over-the-hill joggers.

To make a six-minute story short, I nearly got lapped (in a four-lap race) by a pack of little speedsters, none of whom could have weighed more than 80 pounds.

I mention this more as a warning than as a confession. If you're at all moldy from glory days too far past, enter the athletic world of your offspring with adult wisdom. Skate-boarding, hopscotch, jump rope, tree-climbing, one-on-one basketball—it's tough stuff, fun but not easy. Expect some stiffness, and probably some humiliation. But expect, too, to enjoy every minute of it.

Getting Specific

So what would it really take to have a fitness program with your kids that would satisfy the energy needs of both parties concerned?

We can't answer that specifically because we don't know the age of your children or the logistic constraints you may be up against. You can't be shooting baskets with your teenager after school, after all, if you're working the second shift.

What we can do, however, is give you a good list of activity ideas and let you take it from there. And remember, whatever you may be able to pull together out of this is miles better than nothing at all. As we've said repeatedly in this book, fitness can be a patch quilt of small efforts rather than a blanket of big ones. Whatever you can find the time to do with your kids will feel like a major change if you're currently doing nothing at all.

☐ *Restrict TV time.* It may not sound like an activity, but just wait until you try it. Considerable "wrestling" will ensue, but it's important that you come out on top. Surveys show that the average American child spends more time in front of television over the course of a year than he or she spends at school. This not only amounts to a lot of inactivity, it subjects children to an estimated 10,00 food commercials a year, most of them for junk. If you've ever grocery-shopped with someone younger than about fifteen, you know the effect TV can have. Worse yet, surveys show that kids tend to consume the kinds of foods they see advertised on TV as they're watching TV. A study of the viewing habits of 7,000 children done by the Harvard School of Public Health found that TV and snacking went hand in hand, as did TV and obesity and TV and poor performance in school.

We're not suggesting a TV prohibition, but we are suggesting priorities. Have the kids decide on the programs they want to watch most, and you do the same. About ninety minutes a day per person should probably be the limit.

☐ *Encourage sports.* Whether it's Little League, Pony League, midget football, soccer, swimming, or any number of "semi-sports" that can be played around the house, just say yes. Parental encouragement—but notice we didn't say parental coercion—can be crucial in getting children to make that often difficult first step into athletic life. Do be sensitive, however, because the dangers of being too pushy can match those of not being pushy enough. On the other hand, if Jane or Johnny does not appear to have any athletic interest or talent, that's no reason to throw-in the "sports" towel. The challenge then simply becomes one of changing the towel to a different color. When my older daughter decided after her second week of tennis lessons that life was too short for that degree of humiliation, we canned them and put up a plywood backboard on the garage for her to hit against instead. The backboard gives everyone else in the family a chance to get some fun exercise, too.

☐ *Encourage play.* There are more ways to be athletic than conventional sports. There's everything from Wiffle ball to tumbling, with room for lots of Frisbee, badminton, horseshoes, volleyball, and croquet in between. If your yard is big enough, don't waste it, and by all means participate with your kids whenever possible. Right after dinner is a good time during the summer months because it prevents overeating and boosts calorie-burning. Invite your children's friends to take part, organize tournaments, and, above all, have fun. If you can teach your children that physical activity can be enjoyable, you're teaching them a lesson that's more apt to endure than the lesson of "no pain, no gain." Kids will turn off to that faster than to a bowl of steamed okra.

☐ *Encourage independence and adventure.* When I was thirteen I built a tree house big enough to sleep three comfortably. It had a tin roof and screened sides, and my two brothers and I slept in it every night during the summer for three years. Not only was it good exercise climbing up to and down from our lofty home away from home at least half a dozen times a day, it filled us with excitement and a feeling of adventure, not to mention a sense of independence from the day-to-day turmoil of a seven-child household. If you have the facilities and kids who might welcome the responsibility and sense of freedom that can come from having one's own "apartment," why not suggest and even help them with the construction. It doesn't have to be the kind of luxury suite that I built. Anything that gives them a refuge—and some exercise—will do. Your goal, after all, is to get them away from the video games and TV, not out of your life.

□ *Spring for as much as you can for a swing set.* There's some amazing stuff available, and you do tend to get what you pay for. If you can afford something with monkey bars and a rope swing, you offer your kids a lot more opportunity for exercise than an outfit with swings only. Or if you're handy, you can build something for a lot less money. I can tell you from personal experience that a good swing set does tend to be a good investment. I did a quick survey of friends and neighbors, and the verdict was unanimous that swing sets earn their keep. If you get yourself a good sturdy one, you may find yourself doing some swinging for old-time's sake yourself.

□ *Think of any pool as better than no pool.* Sure, we all dream about the in-ground, but kids usually can have just as much fun—and get almost as much exercise—jumping and splashing in an above-ground pool. The dedicated swimmer of laps is going to be left short, of course, but how many adolescents does that include? And remember again: Your mission is to provide alternatives to the "vegetation" encouraged by the latest computer game or the TV. Even a pool in the price range of $175 and measuring only 3 feet by 12 feet can provide a lot more exercise than a Nintendo game.

□ *Go for nature/litter walks.* In addition to being great exercise, going for walks with your children can be a very special time for interacting with them, and it can be very instructional. Depending on where you live and where you walk, you can discuss either Mother Nature or you can discuss trash. My eight-year-old and I have a lot of fun trying to imagine the types of people responsible for discarding the items we encounter. Fast-food containers, beer cans, and cigarette packs are relatively easy. It's the mattresses, tires, refrigerators, and fully loaded Hefty bags that make us wonder.

17

Fitness in the City: The Taxi Not Taken

Shimer

Stormy, husky, brawling,
City of the big shoulders.
—Carl Sandburg, 1878–1967

You've got a great concept here, gentlemen, but where does it leave the city dweller? How are the nature walks, home repairs, yard work, and gardening going to fit into the life of someone whose sole claim to real estate is the dirt in the pot of ivy on the kitchen sink?"

The question came from our editor, Rick Horgan, and while it seemed on the surface to be a valid one, we had him convinced in short order that opportunities for physical activity are not only more prevalent in an urban setting, they're more intrinsically practical. We offered the following hypothetical examples of two American families to make our point. The Millers live on four acres outside the small town of Hugo, Oklahoma, while the Albrights live in an apartment on the Upper West Side in New York. It's ten o'clock on a typical Saturday morning in May.

Mrs. Miller: "What do you kids have planned for today?"

Mat, age fourteen: "Jason got a new computer game for his birthday. Could you drop me off if I can get a ride back?"

Susan, age twelve: "The new Tom Hanks movie is at the mall. Will you pick me up if Melissa's mom can take us?"

Mrs. Miller, as usual, agrees to both trips.

Mrs. Albright: "What do you kids have planned for today?"

104

Robert, age fourteen: "Our science teacher told us there's a new boa constricter at the zoo. Is it all right if Andy Jenkins and I check it out, and maybe stop at the park on the way back?"

Angela, age twelve: "Tina and I have to go to the library to work on our history report. Is it okay if we do some shopping at Macy's on the way?"

Mrs. Albright also gives her okay.

Get the picture? The "great outdoors" have the Millers burning gasoline while the "convenience" of city life has the Albrights burning calories. And the scenario doesn't stop with the kids. Mrs. Miller on that Saturday decides to drive to see a friend between dropping off Matt and picking up Susan. Mrs. Albright, on the other hand, decides to join a friend for a walk to the Metropolitan Museum of Art.

And the men of the houses?

Mr. Miller spends one hour riding his lawn tractor and another hour riding his Harley Davidson. Mr. Albright spends three hours playing softball in Central Park.

Fine, you say, the Albrights get frisky on Saturdays, but only because they're caged like animals all week.

Sorry, but the Albright children walk six blocks to and from school each day, which is about a mile round trip, and Mrs. Albright has adopted a new "no cabs allowed" policy that has added an average of 2 miles a day of legwork to her life. And Mr. Albright—in addition to walking four blocks to and from the subway each day—has become, by his own admission, a "stair-aholic." Unless he is running ridiculously late, he will avoid both elevators and escalators as if they were as bad for his heart as one of those grilled sausages from a vendor on 42nd Street.

The Albrights, in short, have managed to make their weekdays as well as their weekends in the city very physical indeed. Compared to the Millers, they live like pioneers, in fact. They walk more, climb more stairs, and engage in more sports. And their physiques reflect their more active lifestyles. Each of the Albrights weighs slightly less than the national average for their age and height, while each of the Millers weighs about 10 percent more.

Beginning to get the point? Yes, we've exaggerated our comparison somewhat for the purpose of contrast, but any urban dweller who has ever complained that opportunities for physical activity are lacking in the urban environment had better forever hold his peace. Cities are veritable gymnasiums of potential activity. As a friend and former neighbor of mine in rural Coopersburg, Pennsylvania, told me about a year after moving to center city Philadelphia, "I haven't had to jog a step since I've been here. The amount of walking I do in an average day is absolutely incredible."

Granted, Larry is extremely cheap, but maybe more of us should be so cheap when saving money can mean burning calories. A cab ride in most major American cities costs about $3.00 per mile. Compare that to the 80 to 100 calories that the average person burns by briskly walking a mile, and those cab dollars begin to make very little sense very quickly. Larry has determined that for every pound of fat he has lost by walking —and he has lost 10 since making his city move—he has saved over $100 in cab fare. Considering all the weight-reduction programs out there that cost money, I think Larry has stepped into a pretty smart deal.

When I asked him how he managed to fit so much "footage" into his busy schedule—he's a writer and editor for *Philadelphia* magazine—he said the first thing he did was to sell his car. He admits it wasn't easy, but now he doesn't miss it at all. If he needs to travel out of town, he rents something big and fancy. Otherwise his "wheels" are his feet. He hoofs about a mile (twelve blocks) to and from work each day, weather permitting, and he tries to walk for at least thirty minutes during his lunch break.

"It's fun because it lets me try a lot of different restaurants," he told me. "It also keeps me from overeating. I'm not going to go ordering prime rib and a couple of scotches knowing I've got a fifteen-minute hike back to the office. Sometimes I'll even pack a lunch and walk down to the waterfront at Penn's Landing and eat as I watch the ships come in."

Larry was especially interested to hear that his postmeal walking boosts the "thermic" effect of his lunches to about 20 percent, a boost that means 20 percent of the calories he eats get burned simply because he eats and walks, rather than walking on an empty stomach.

Stepping Up to Better Health

But opportunities for horizontal ambulation aside, city life also offers countless chances to travel vertically. Where else, short of a Mayan ruin, are you going to find the concentration of stairs that you can find in any major city today? The high-rise profile of the American city has been the result of sky-high real estate prices, unfortunately, but why look a gift horse in the mouth? Stairs remain one of the last great "natural" exercise opportunities available to modern man. All we need to do is, like Mr. Albright, learn to look at elevators and escalators as environmental hazards as blatant as the street vendor's sausage: Take one and you shorten your life. That may sound a little drastic, but not when considering the stair-climbing calculations mentioned earlier—each step taken adds about four seconds to your life. Think about that the next time you're feeling life is too short to be waiting for an elevator.

Other interesting arithmetic on the benefits of stair-climbing comes from a variety of sources. A study done by an insurance company in Finland found that a "significant level of fitness" was achieved by people who climbed an average of twenty-five flights of stairs a day. This sounds like a lot, but it's not if you break it into small bouts and include stair-climbing in your mini-walks. But beware of tackling too many flights at any one time, because the degree of exertion escalates rather quickly. Research shows that a stair-climber's heart rate goes up as much as 10 beats for every flight climbed.

The potential for vigorous exercise is there, but that's not why we recommend stair-climbing. It's a great calorie burner regardless of how fast you go. Nor is coming down any cake walk—the energy cost is about 40 percent of the price of going up.

Health and Wealth = The Taxi Not Taken

Walking makes so much sense from so many angles that we thought we'd leave you with this chart. The figures will be less dramatic if your usual form of transportation is bus or subway, but even those fares can begin to mount up over the years—just like the pounds of fat that they're perpetuating.

Calories burned per block (based on 12 blocks per mile)	7
Blocks walked per day	24 (about 2 miles)
Calories burned per day	168
Calories burned per year	61,320
Amount of potential fat loss due to 61,320 calories expended per year	17.5 pounds
Amount of money saved in cab fares per year	$1,934.50

(based on 1989 rates in New York City, assuming trips are of 1 mile each)

18

Fitness for the Obese

Stamford

He that hath patience can compass anything.
—François Rabelais, 1483–1553

Exercise physiology became my life's work and I grew up to be fit and muscular, but along the way there were changes in my physique that rival the best of ugly duckling stories. I wasn't fat enough to be the butt of jokes in grade school, but I was fat enough never to take my shirt off in public, even on the hottest days. Maybe that's why I was able to escape ridicule. I was self-conscious enough about my weight to keep it under cover. By the sixth grade, however, that was becoming difficult. I was wearing a pair of 36-inch-waist pants, snugly. At some point, just being self-conscious wasn't going to be enough. That point came in junior high.

Girls entered the picture, and suddenly I *did* want to be noticed. It was time for battle. A hundred sit-ups every morning before breakfast. Push-ups, pull-ups, and workouts with resistance springs and barbells after school. The change I achieved in a year was dramatic. And I was hooked.

But I was hooked on more than just exercise, I learned. I was hooked on the belief that if I could do it, anybody could. My sympathy for the obese disappeared along with my potbelly. People were fat simply because they ate too much and exercised too little. If they really wanted to change, all they had to do was whip themselves into shape the way I had. And the more I learned about the calorie-burning effects of exercise, the more my prejudice grew. People who were overweight were merely victims of their own sloth. But then I met Margaret.

Margaret was a plump older woman who used to go for walks in my old neighborhood, usually late in the day under the cover of twilight. Frequently, I would pass her on my evening runs, but because she was going like the tortoise and I like the hare, I never felt the need to blurt much more than a breathy "Hi." One evening we met face to face, however, as I was walking to cool down from my run, and so suddenly that we had the obligation to do more than just exchange hellos. She appeared very timid, almost frightened. I was basking self-righteously in the aftermath of my 5-mile jaunt, so I took the initiative by remarking that it was nice to meet someone else interested in fitness. I could see right away she sensed my insincerity, but she wasn't about to nail me for it. She simply thanked me. But she was certainly not a "fitness buff" like me, she said. No, she was just another "fatso" doing too little too late to try to slim down.

I agreed, of course, but I couldn't let her know that. I kept my phoniness going by telling her not to be so hard on herself, that she was doing what was "right for her," but said maybe she might try some slow jogging sometime to speed her weight loss. After explaining who I was, I even gave her some specific instructions on pace and distance. She seemed thankful if not enthusiastic, and we parted pleasantly. Would my advice have an effect?

A week went by. No Margaret.

Two weeks went by. No Margaret.

More than a month passed before I saw Margaret out on the trail again, so of course I asked her where she had been. It seems she had taken my advice. She had listened to the "exercise expert" and tried mixing some jogging into her walks. And she had wound up with severe shin pain and a bruised heel for her efforts. Only now, after five weeks, was she feeling back to normal enough to resume her former schedule.

Nice job, *Doctor* Stamford.

But if you can believe it, our relationship improved greatly after that day. I had been humbled, which no doubt helped things from her perspective, but it seemed to help me, too. For the first time since my childhood, I began to develop a sensitivity for the burdens that obesity can impose. We got to know each other better in the weeks that followed, well enough for Margaret to confess that she actually used to hate to see me coming.

"Here he comes again. Mr. Macho-Health. He probably laughs it up with all his super-fit buddies about the fatty who moves like a wounded turtle."

She had it just about right, and it embarrassed me. But it also taught me a darned good lesson. It taught me—and also reminded me—of the mental as well as physical stresses obesity can inflict. How had I gotten so high on my horse? Just because I had been able to endure a year of torturous weight loss and was able to continue in the grueling vigilance it took to maintain that weight loss, did that give me the right to sneer at mortals like Margaret?

I'm sorry, Margaret, and I'm sorry to all the others like you who may have been chagrined by my insensitivity. And I'm sorry, too, for the aerobic principles that encouraged my callousness. "Get them up, get them moving, get them sweating. Forget that they may be embarrassed, in discomfort, or feeling depressed. The aerobic elixir will work its magic cure."

The past twenty years stand as testimony to the errors in that way of thinking. Obesity in the United States is at an all-time high among adults and children alike. It's time we gave the Margarets of the world the special consideration they deserve.

Fat Bodies, Thin Egos

Why has the fitness movement done such a poor job of helping the obese? Let's count the ways:

1. People who are obese feel conspicuous enough in public. Few relish calling even more attention to themselves by showcasing their physical limitations through exercise.
2. People who are obese have trouble enough performing the basic activities of daily living, much less the rigorous movements required by aerobic workouts. Jogging can be especially disheartening for the overweight.
3. People who are obese have trouble dissipating body heat, which can cause considerable discomfort when strenuous exercise is attempted.
4. People who are obese may experience uncomfortable and even dangerous strain on the heart during heavy exertion as excess fat in the area of the chest and upper abdomen can offer unnatural resistance to heart movement. Excess fat can hinder breathing as well, by causing undue pressure on the lungs and muscles of the diaphragm.
5. People who are obese tend to lack the self-esteem it takes to embark on an aerobic exercise program in the first place.

Obesity might not make aerobic exercise hopeless, in other words, but it can sure make it feel hapless. Simple physical activity, on the other hand—basic movement involved in around-the-house chores, light sporting activities, and walking—can burn calories *without extinguishing motivation.*

Of vital importance, too, is getting dietary fats out of the diet, because they're the building blocks of body fat in the first place. Reducing sugar in the diet also is important, as is reducing meal size while increasing meal frequency. We'll be talking more about all three of these dietary strategies in the next section of this book, but trust for the time being that the end result is a crucial one: fewer fat molecules in the bloodstream and a reduced tendency for those molecules to be snatched up by fat cells for storage. Combine these strategies with more fiber in the diet, which also can reduce fat absorption while at the same time providing feelings of fullness, and you've got as good a fat-fighting plan as you're going to get. It might not pull the pounds off as fast as some of the medically unsound "crash" programs can, but for reasons we'll also be examining in our diet section, consider that a plus rather than a minus. *The longer weight loss takes, the longer it tends to last.* Feel free to etch that in stone somewhere, or at least write it on your refrigerator if you think it'll help. Haste makes waste in the world of weight loss just as it does everywhere else.

But more on the dietary aspects of life-long fat loss later. Here are the ground rules for getting the physical side of fat loss started.

□ *Go soft and slow.* The mistake many overweight people make is that they start so fast they trip just getting out of the gate. Start slowly and start comfortably. Do not make the mistake of discouraging yourself unnecessarily. You're a big person, so movement is going to involve effort. There's a rosy side to that, however, in that you burn more calories for any given task you undertake. Someone who weighs 130 pounds burns about 350 calories in an hour of mowing grass. Someone who weighs 200 burns nearly 200 calories an hour more.

□ *Stop and go.* Do a little, then rest a little. Calorie-burning doesn't have to be continuous to count. Above all, avoid extreme exhaustion. If you have high blood pressure, which many overweight people do, extreme exhaustion could be dangerous. Besides, you burn more calories being active for thirty minutes out of sixty than by needing to call it quits after only fifteen.

□ *Keep cool.* Because you are, in fact, well "insulated," keeping cool is going to be harder for you than for people of normal weight. But don't despair. Air-conditioned shopping malls can be great for cool walks, or you can make efforts to restrict outdoor activity to early morning and twilight hours. Avoid bright sunlight at all cost because it can make you uncomfortable via radiant heat even though air temperature may be fairly low. High humidity is even worse than bright sunlight, because it discourages the cooling process associated with the evaporation of sweat. Combine the two—bright sunlight and high humidity—and you've got an inferno best avoided entirely. As for dress, go loose and go natural. Loose-fitting clothing allows air to circulate over the skin and can actually fan you as it flaps. Natural fabrics are superior to synthetics because they allow a greater escape of body heat. *Never* wear a rubber sweat suit. You've already got more insulation than you need.

☐ *Take to the water.* Because fat is more buoyant than muscle, water can boost your feelings of physical prowess. Don't feel you need to swim laps for exercise, however. Fun water sports such as water polo or even just splashing around can burn calories, too.

☐ *Get some activity sitting down.* Cycling also is a good activity option for the obese because the bike, and not you, supports your poundage. Go easy, however, because cycling can be demanding. And don't forget to keep it fun and/or practical.

A trick I use to get myself to use my bike more is to think about the greenhouse effect. Why burn gas and money to pollute the air when with my bike I can burn just calories?

☐ *Weigh the pros and cons of partnership.* An activity partner can be helpful if he or she shares your levels of both fitness and commitment. If not, you could have an anchor on your hands when you're already pulling enough weight as it is. Or if the person is more fit than you, you could have too tough an act to follow. Unless the partner you can find is a near perfect one, you might be better off going it alone.

☐ *Be flexible.* By being flexible you'll have less of a tendency to break. This applies to your commitments to diet as well as to physical activity. Personally, I use what I call the 80/20 Rule. Eighty percent of the time I'm good, and I don't worry about the 20 percent of the time I'm bad. The mistake a lot of us make is that we try to be perfect, which only leaves us filled with self-loathing when we fall short. Don't put that pressure on yourself. Forget perfection, just be good.

☐ *Don't rely on willpower.* If you're having to resort to willpower to build activity into your life, there's something wrong with the activity. This goes for dietary changes, too. Willpower implies an element of conflict, which it would be better to resolve. Your goal should be to win yourself over with as little force as possible.

☐ *Declare war on boredom.* What usually calls upon willpower most? Yes, the "B" word. Don't let it happen. Be imaginative enough to fit physical activity into your life in ways that do not feel oppressively mindless.

☐ *Make physical activity "necessary."* Think about throwing away the remote control channel changer or selling the ride-on lawn mower, weed-trimmer, or leaf-blower. Maybe unplug the electric clothes dryer for six months out of the year. These may sound like drastic moves, but are they any more drastic than attempting to stick to a three-workouts-a-week aerobic exercise schedule? We think not.

A Word on "Crashing" It Off

When I speak before a group, the most often asked question is my opinion about the latest weight-loss fad. There have been many in recent years, but they all have a few things in common.

First, they break all rules of common sense. Second, they promote water and muscle loss, and lost inches occur because tissues become dehydrated. Third, they result in little fat loss unless the program is combined with lots of physical activity. Fourth, no new and worthwhile lifestyle habits are developed. And fifth, the long-range success rate is near zero.

With that said, however, I must admit that some severely overweight people have had success with extreme weight-loss regimens offered under medical supervision. These plans usually call for three liquid meals a day that offer very few calories but do supply required nutrients. On the best of these programs, a considerable amount of walking, however, also is advised. Two friends of mine are stars of one such program run by a local hospital, he having lost more than 100 pounds and she more than 50. There was nothing magical about their success, however. He walked 8 to 12 miles a day, while she walked 4 to 6. My friends are now on the "maintenance" phase of this plan, which involves a very low-fat diet while continuing their long, comfortable daily walks. They are, in short, following the tenents of this book.

Could my friends have gotten to where they are now without taking the drastic steps they did?

Maybe not. Maybe without immersing themselves to that degree, they would have lost interest along the way. We'll never know for sure. We do know, however, that they're comfortable and happy with the lifestyle they're leading now.

My point?

Give moderation a try before you go to extremes. Give it a good try, however—six months at least. If you're not happy with your results, then consider more drastic measures.

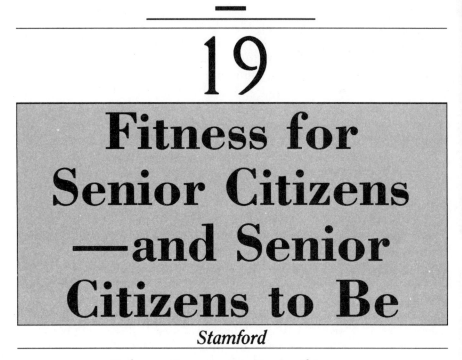

19

Fitness for Senior Citizens —and Senior Citizens to Be

Stamford

*To be seventy years young is something
far more cheerful than to be forty years old.*
—Oliver Wendell Holmes, 1809–1894

We call them the "golden years," the best years—the ones we work for, the ones that will make it all worthwhile. Gone will be the worry, the scrimping to make payments, the arguments with the children, and the conflicts at work. Just peace of mind, good books, great vacations, and well-behaved grandchildren bouncing on our knees.

Or so we hope. So we start planning for our golden years as early as possible with pension plans, Keoghs, and IRAs. But guess what. Our golden years will be gruesome years if we don't make efforts to preserve ourselves physically as well as financially. The Cadillac will be driven by your son-in-law if all you can drive is a wheelchair, and Uncle George will be the one with his feet up at your beachfront condo if your R and R is being taken in a hospital.

It's not fun to think about, but it can happen.

"But I've been living like this my entire life. What difference is it really going to make if I change now?"

That's a frequently asked question with a very important answer. Unhealthy living becomes more unhealthful with every passing day. The body's defenses against bad health habits begin to weaken naturally with age, but they also begin to weaken from the repeated abuse of the bad habits themselves. Combine the two and you've got double trouble. A hedonistic senior citizen is a time bomb whose clock ticks faster with each and every abuse.

Sound scary?

It should. Whether the offense is tobacco, alcohol abuse, a high-fat diet, or a totally sedentary lifestyle, it's going to be worse for you tomorrow than it is today. Think of your body as a chain, and think of the aging process as the force that eventually will find the chain's weakest link. Bad health habits are chisels tapping away at some of the most vital links in that chain, links that are being given a tough enough time by the meddlings of Father Time.

We'll be looking at the effects of bad habits in closer detail later in Part IV, but the point we wish to stress here is simply that our retirement years should not be taken sitting down. We might even think of them as years we need to "get in shape for" if we're going to escape their hazards. That might seem a little unfair if you've worked hard all your life and look forward to a virtual "life of Riley," but how much fun can such a life be if you become paralyzed by a stroke or need to be confined to a wheelchair because of softening of the bones?

When I propose scenarios like that to people of retirement age, I often get the same reaction. They say that the hard work they've done all their lives will carry them through, that the very labor they're retiring from will give them the strength to coast through retirement unscathed.

Research doesn't agree, and the message is clear. An active lifestyle must be a companion for life in order to be protective against cardiovascular disease. Studies show that well-trained athletes who became sedentary after their days of competition enjoy no greater immunity from heart attacks or strokes than men who have been sedentary their entire lives. Total inactivity is something our bodies were not designed to handle. Loss of both muscle and bone can begin in less than a week as a result of total bed rest, so why should we expect days spent doing nothing more strenuous than crossword puzzles to be much kinder?

When an older person fails to engage in adequate physical movement, muscles wither and joints lose mobility. The eventual result can be that movement becomes not just difficult but prohibitively painful, thus discouraging activity even further and setting into motion a very deleterious cycle.

It'll never happen to you, you say? You'll be able to sense infirmity like that coming on years ahead of time?

Don't be so sure. Aging leads to a decline in muscle mass, flexibility, and aerobic capacity in its own right, but magnify the decline by retiring to a totally sedentary lifestyle and the process can be accelerated greatly. If you don't think so, consider all the things you cannot do now that you could do easily at age twenty. What's to make you think the years ahead are going to be any kinder? They're going to be even tougher. And don't think the miracles of modern medicine will be there to bail you out. Medical advances may be able to help you live long, but keeping physically active enough to have the strength to live well is going to be your job. Longer life for anyone not willing to keep in shape for it could wind up being less of a blessing than a curse. Is "golden" really the word to describe years spent alive thanks to medical technology, and yet disabled because we didn't see fit to prepare for those extra years?

The Other Side of the Hill Doesn't Have to Be a Cliff

But enough bad news and enough scoldings. The good news is that the physical declines associated with aging, though they can't be halted, can be slowed. We age for a variety of very complex reasons, all of which wind up being influenced, however, by two factors very much within our control: physical activity and diet. As we mentioned, the body's physical capacities—muscular strength, flexibility, aerobic capacity, and even skeletal strength and hand-eye coordination—all tend to decline as a natural consequence of the aging process. Much of the decline, however, is due to a reduction in physical activity, which is our decision and not Father Time's. Research leaves no doubt that all of the systems mentioned remain far better preserved in people who remain active into their twilight years.

But something else of vital importance happens when people stay active into old age: They give themselves the opportunity to eat more and hence take in more vital nutrients without getting fat. Physical activity carried into middle and old age not only burns calories in its own right, it helps to slow the decline in muscle mass, which in turn helps to keep the body burning calories at a more youthful rate even while at rest. Studies show that muscle tissue, pound for pound, burns many more calories than fat even as the muscle tissue lies dormant, so of course maintaining muscle is going to be a sizable advantage for anyone fighting the battle of the bulge, regardless of age.

More muscle tissue for seniors appears to be especially critical, however, because of the extra caloric leeway it allows. Most older people take in about 20 percent fewer calories—a natural response to their reduced muscle mass and lower activity levels—but there is nothing natural about the 20 percent drop in vitamins, minerals, and protein this includes. Even though our needs for calories drop with age, our needs for nutrients remain as youthful as ever—and may even increase due to reduced absorption by our aging digestive tracts.

Physical activity to the rescue: Increased physical activity allows more calories to be consumed, and hence more nutrients, but without weight gain as a result.

But something else can allow more nutrients to be consumed—less fat. Reducing fat calories, which tend to be empty ones, can allow for more calories to come from complex carbohydrates and low-fat proteins which, calorie for calorie, are much richer in nutrients. Feel free to flip ahead to our nutrition section if you're curious about the exact foods we recommend, but it's our guess that you know them already: complex carbohydrates (potatoes, bread, pastas, cereals), low-fat proteins (baked or broiled chicken and fish, beans, low-fat dairy products), and all the fresh fruits and vegetables you can eat. Maybe you've been presented a similar list at some point by your doctor. A diet that centers on nutritious, low-fat foods can allow you your full stomach—and a relatively flat stomach, too. And this, of course, applies whether you're eight or eighty.

Getting Started

But now it's time to talk turkey to those of you who are already senior citizens. And maybe just the thought of embarking on a "health kick" at this stage of your life has raised your heart rate.

Relax. Fitness does not have to mean the kind of heart-pumping efforts that you have been conditioned to believe. You can do it your way—slowly, peacefully, pleasantly. Don't let the word "exercise" even cross your mind. Simply think movement, movement that's going to preserve muscle mass and skeletal strength and flexibility in the joints. And if it's of any help, think of the "exercise" routines that helped keep Pablo Picasso or Arthur Fiedler so well preserved. For Picasso it was wielding nothing heavier than a paint brush, and for Fiedler a conductor's baton. Just think of what you can do with a walking stick, pair of hedge clippers, or perhaps a paint brush or musical instrument of your own. Don't think intensity at your age, think joy.

And above all, realize that it really is "never too late." I've been a firm believer of that ever since doing a series of studies with elderly mental patients as a graduate student in exercise physiology some twenty years ago. To challenge the prevailing notion at the time that at least a minimally active background was necessary for someone to make appreciable fitness gains late in life, I worked with a group of elderly patients who had been restricted to a state hospital since early childhood. I started them out with very leisurely walking on a motorized treadmill, and within just a few months the improvement in their fitness levels was phenomenal. It seemed almost as though their physical potential had been waiting all those years to blossom. They weren't over the hill. Far from it. They had never even been given a chance to approach their peak.

Could it be time for you to approach yours?

The Game Plan

☐ *Start with a checkup.* Tell your doctor you plan to increase the physical activity in your life, giving an idea of what you have in mind, and request to be checked out accordingly. If it involves a blood test or even an exercise stress test, don't hesitate. Better safe than sorry.

☐ *Establish a working relationship with your doctor.* Announce that you've decided to embark on a health-improvement program and ask for your doctor's help. It can be a valuable boost knowing you've got the approval and even encouragement of the medical establishment.

☐ *Reevaluate your medications.* If you take blood pressure medication, for example, don't stop, but do keep in mind that by reducing the fat in your diet and being more active, you may be able to reduce your dosage and possibly even discontinue your medication altogether. Don't even think about such changes, however, without the full approval of your doctor.

☐ *Start small and be in no hurry.* Millions of senior citizens watched the aerobic bandwagon race by, and for good reason: It was simply moving too fast. Your goal should be to burn at least 150 calories, and up to 300 calories a day above the 1,500 to 1,800 or so that you would burn simply by reading or watching TV. How you choose to burn those calories is totally up to you, although the chart we presented in chapter 12 might give you some ideas. Whatever you decide on, don't make it burdensome. You'll grow to resent the activity and eventually abandon it if it causes you stress. Which brings us to perhaps our most important tip of all. . . .

☐ *Put a premium on pleasure.* You are retired, after all. You've paid your dues. It's time to engage in physical activity for the sheer joy of it. Consider gardening, light carpentry projects, bird-watching, fishing—anything that lets you feel youthful and alive. What you want to avoid are activities that feel toilsome. You've had your fill of that. As Joseph Campbell said, "Seek your bliss." You have earned the right.

☐ *Don't be afraid to exercise your creativity.* A hobby or craft such as painting, sculpturing, or pottery might not seem like much exercise, but compared to reading the obituaries, it's like a jog in the park. Check with the colleges or universities in your area. Many have programs that invite seniors to spend time on campus taking classes of special interest at little or no cost. And remember: Anything that gets you on your feet and out of the house is exercise. And if it gets your mind working, better yet. There's more to health, after all, than just the body. There's the mental enthusiasm it takes to want to keep active.

☐ *"Work out" with your grandchildren.* If you've got some and they're nearby, don't waste them. Depending on their age, they can be very uplifting companions in a wide variety of activities ranging from walks to fishing expeditions to simple maintenance chores around the house. You'll find they can help keep your wits in shape, as well.

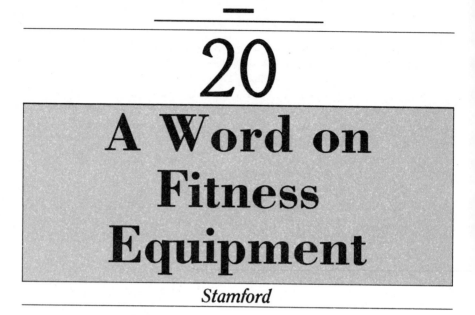

20

A Word on Fitness Equipment

Stamford

*We are becoming the servants . . . of
the machines we have created to serve us.*
—John Kenneth Galbraith, 1908–

If our assault on aerobic exercise has seemed thus far to come down especially hard on fitness equipment, we should make some amends, because fitness equipment can have a place in the health strategy we propose. For city dwellers who'd rather not take to the streets, for the obese who'd rather not burn their calories in public, for the elderly who may not be capable of getting outdoors, and for anyone faced with bad weather, a stationary bike or rowing machine can answer the call.

Our dissatisfaction with fitness equipment has not been with the equipment itself, you see, only with how it's been used, which has been hatefully, rarely, or never.

But has that been the fault of the equipment?

No, it's been the fault of the aerobic doctrine's telling us how to use it. We have been told to go for at least twenty to thirty minutes at a stretch, and we've been told to maintain a substantially elevated "target" heart rate. No wonder the stuff collects dust. In my twenty years of experience in the fitness field, I can safely say that nothing has created as much initial enthusiasm—or as much eventual disappointment—as fitness machines. I'm going to guess that fewer than 10 percent of all fitness equipment ever purchased has gone on to be used on a regular basis. The stuff gets tried, put aside, and eventually put out of sight, and out of mind, forever.

But again, the fault lies not with the equipment, but rather with the instructions we've been given to use it. Aerobic doctrine made the rowing machine as unsavory as the thirty-minute jog. It's time we gave our fitness hardware a second chance.

How?

By approaching it in the same way Porter and I have been suggesting that other forms of activity be approached—without a sense of obligation, without a master plan, and, above all, without dread. Don't feel you need to put in at least twenty minutes at a time, and don't feel your efforts need to be strenuous. That's what put the device in drydock in the first place, remember? Your attitude should be merely to use the device for however long and however often feels convenient. Exercise gotten in this "piece by peace" way can do everything that continuous, aerobic exercise can do in helping to promote human health. This holds especially true for those who have been avoiding physical activity altogether. The resounding message to come from the latest fitness research has been that the greatest health gains stand to be enjoyed by people who go from being totally sedentary to at least moderately active. Whether aerobic fitness is achieved or not, huge rewards await the couch potato who's willing simply to pull him- or herself up out of the upholstery. For example:

You've got five minutes to kill while the casserole is cooking in the microwave?

Spend it on the stationary bike, and without feeling you need to break a sweat.

Need something to do while the bathtub fills?

Squeeze in twenty strokes on the rowing machine.

Feel like clobbering your nine-year-old?

Unleash your energy on that pricey ski machine, instead.

Get the picture? Spare moments can be turned into health-making moments if intensity and duration can be forgotten. Simply look at any time you spend with your fitness equipment as better than no time at all.

Which fitness devices lend themselves to this sort of approach best?

Any device that's conveniently located, first of all. Step one in giving fitness equipment a second chance is to place it where it can be used. If five minutes is all you have, you don't want to be spending three of those minutes getting a device out of a closet and then putting it away again, and you don't want to be trooping out to the garage, either. You may need to swallow your decorative pride here a bit, but it can be well worth it for your health. If you've got a stationary bike or rowing machine, keep it where you'll use it. Barbells, ski machines, and treadmills, too. Don't let simple distance or inconvenience come between you and the stuff that really can help improve your physique, your attitude, and your odds of a longer life.

As for what to use, you shouldn't even be asking that question if you've already got the device of your dreams stowed away somewhere. Get it out. Apologize to it. Promise it a new start.

If you don't already have a fitness device, however, you'll want to ask yourself two questions: What sort of device do you see as being most pleasurable to use, and what sort of money are you willing to spend?

People who are considerably overweight generally do better on stationary bicycles than rowing machines, if that's any help. And as for the cash question—don't scrimp. If you're serious about this device, which you should be, then put your money where your heart is. You should expect to spend in the neighborhood of $300 for a stationary bike or rowing machine, and between $400 and $700 for a ski machine or treadmill.

You can certainly go higher on all of these devices, of course, and don't let us be the ones to stop you. If you honestly think that making a commitment financially will help you make a commitment physically, be our guest. At the risk of doing some advertising, there are some very worthwhile and durable devices out there. Porter tells me he has a Schwinn Aer-Dyne stationary bicycle that turned 20,000 miles not long ago, and I've heard good things about some of the more expensive rowing machines. (You might want to be wary of a rowing machine if you suffer from low back trouble, however, as they can stress the low back muscles more than might be comfortable.)

Are we "selling out" by allowing room for fitness equipment in our *Fitness Without Exercise* message?

We don't think so. Exercise is exercise only if it feels like exercise, only if it's onerous, burdensome, and dreadful. If a piece of fitness equipment can be used in a spontaneous and even enjoyable way, it gets our stamp of approval. Only if it begins to own you should you begin to worry. The activity in your life should serve you, after all, not enslave you. Any device that does that *should* be part of your next garage sale.

NUTRITION AND WEIGHT CONTROL: EAT BETTER, WEIGH LESS

21

The Answer to the Riddle of the Expanding American: F.A.T.

Shimer

You deserve a break today.
—The McDonald's Corporation

It didn't bother me that he was ahead of me in the express lane at the supermarket with at least twenty items when the limit was ten, and I could even accept the nutritional absurdity of what he was buying. A jar of marshmallow sauce, beer, bologna, cream cheese, a pound of butter, and a bag of Oreo cookies stick in my mind. What got me was the jogging suit and the potbelly.

Where had this guy missed the point? Didn't he realize that not even a jog to the moon could do much good against a diet like that?

I was still thinking about this "jogger" as I drove home with my carrots, low-fat yogurt, and tuna packed in water. Maybe he hadn't missed the point. Maybe the point simply had never been well enough made. There were certainly no strong dietary warnings in any of the best-selling running books. Jim Fixx at one point claimed that "running provides at least a partial refuge from contemporary dietary pressure . . . to eat wisely."

Such inducement was all that millions of runners needed to start looking at junk food as the staples of performance-boosting "carbo-loads." Maybe that was it. Maybe this guy in the supermarket, potbelly and all, was getting ready for a big race.

The absurdity of it all was just beginning to sink in when an ad came on the radio that put the icing on the cake. A local diner was offering something it called its "late night breakfast special": two eggs, choice of bacon or sausage, "home-fried" potatoes (how they managed that at the diner, I don't know), two pancakes "heaped" with butter, and unlimited refills on coffee. Normally priced at $3.49, the feast was being offered for an eye-opening $2.29 after 10:00 P.M. Just the thing for a case of the munchies after a night of beer drinking, I thought to myself.

When I got home, I ran the "late night breakfast special" through some calculations. As I suspected, it was a nightmare in terms of both calories and fat. The meal came to 1,240 calories, nearly two-thirds of them from fat. Granted, there are a fair number of shift workers in the area where I live who could have been coming to the late night breakfast special as their "morning" meal, but even so, anything that's two-thirds fat is wrong for any time of the day. And it certainly is no way to prepare for bed. Weight gain aside, eating a high-fat meal even within several hours of retiring can substantially increase risks of both heart attack and stroke. The danger arises from clots that can form in the blood. Fats entering the bloodstream from a high-fat meal literally can make the blood "sticky," which can be especially dangerous when blood flow slows during the sleep process. For someone with partially blocked arteries, the late night supper could be the last.

And yet late night eating is as American as the refrigerator. If we're not chowing down to a fat-laden fast-food meal, we're fixing something at home to help us turn out the lights. No wonder the aerobics movement hasn't been able to put even a dent in the growing problem of obesity in this country. Four out of ten American adults currently weigh at least 20 percent more than is thought to be optimal for good health. That comes to roughly 2.5 billion pounds of excess body fat—the weight of approximately 300,000 adult hippos. Where's our sense of pride?

It's alive, but it's not well. Surveys suggest that as many as one-third of us may be engaged in a weight-loss effort as you read this. Fully 90 percent, however, will fail. Is it that we lack the willpower to lose weight?

No. We lack the patience. We'll try anything that promises to pay off quickly, but we'll balk at a plan that admits to taking some time. And yet weight loss must take time. That's the only way it can work. There's a Golden Rule to weight loss that should be written on the bathroom scale of anyone who's really serious about losing weight: *The faster pounds come off, the more likely they are to return*—with interest! This is true for metabolic reasons, but it's also true for psychological ones. Any dietary program that shocks the body is going to shock the mind. And with shock comes recoil. The mistake most dieters make is that they embark on a journey that is so uncomfortable that of course they're going to jump ship. The secret is to implement change slowly, almost imperceptibly. Struggle is a forecast of defeat.

Calories Are Not the Problem

Why has the American waistline been guilty of such rapid expansion. Is it gluttony, plain and simple? Eating too much, too often—the "late night breakfast special" and that jogger's express lane "snack" foods being prime examples?

No, simple gluttony is not our only problem. This may surprise you, but the average American today does not consume more calories than in 1910. So how can it be that we weigh, on average, about 10 percent more than in 1910?

The fitness movement would like to put the blame squarely on the shoulders of "reduced physical activity," but to do so misses some critical points. There have been dietary changes that have occurred over the past eighty years that have had as much to do with the change in the cut of the American jib as less physical activity. Specifically:

- Our intake of dietary fat has increased by about 15 percent.
- Our intake of refined sugar has risen by about 20 percent.
- We have moved toward eating large, infrequent meals as opposed to smaller meals spaced more evenly throughout the day.

Add the fact that many of us now look to food as much for reducing stress as for providing nourishment, and you've got a dream come true for the biochemical as well as psychological processes of which obesity is made. We eat with the wrong *frequency*, the wrong *attitude*, and the *types* of food we eat are wrong. Put the three together and you've got F.A.T.— literally as well as figuratively. The combination is so conducive to weight gain that amount, as measured by actual calories consumed, becomes relatively unimportant. Millions of Americans remain overweight despite caloric intakes that are not out of line with their needs. It's the combination of F.A.T. that's conspiring to keep them plump. Even with the addition of an aerobic exercise program, F.A.T. can prevent weight loss. Let's consider the case of Barbara to get a closer look at why the F.A.T. combination is so "inflationary." Feel free to identify where appropriate.

Frequency

Barbara would like to lose 20 pounds, so she has only coffee for breakfast and "just a salad" for lunch. This allows her to feel she well deserves her 1,200-calorie dinner of roast beef with gravy, mashed potatoes with butter, creamed corn, and chocolate ice cream. Little does Barbara realize, however, that this pattern of eating, even though her calories are not excessive, is thwarting her weight-loss efforts in two very critical ways.

First, by eating so much at one sitting, Barbara is causing her pancreas to release proportionately more insulin than would be called upon by a smaller meal, the result being that the calories she consumes are more likely to be stored as fat than burned for energy.

Second, the size of Barbara's meal is going to leave her feeling un-inclined to do much more than wrestle with the evening paper the rest of the night, the result being that she will be deprived of the opportunity to capitalize on a calorie-burning phenomenon known as the Thermic Effect of Exercise. If Barbara would just go for a short walk, cut some grass, or even just run the vacuum cleaner, she would not only benefit from the calorie-burning of these activities in and of themselves, but she would be adding at least 10 percent to their calorie-burning simply by virtue of doing them with food in her stomach. The explanation is a complicated one, but what it boils down to is that physical activity brings oxygen into the body in a way that helps food burn slightly "hotter," and dietary fats especially. Exercising shortly before eating can accomplish the same effect, so Barbara could enjoy a greater caloric burn from her meal if she were to be moderately active prior to eating as well as after. (More on the digestive effects of moderate activity later in this section.)

The above two factors—an oversized meal and accompanying in-activity—if seemingly trivial, are not. Research shows that many people who are obese eat less than people of normal weight but make the mistake, like Barbara, of skipping meals to be able to eat one big one. In one study, fully 80 percent of the obese people surveyed were eating less than people of normal weight but were making Barbara's "one big meal a day" mistake. Big meals tend to produce big waistlines. Think of the issue in those simple terms if you think it'll help.

Attitude

But what motivates the "one-big-meal-a-day" eating pattern in the first place?

Some of us are simply all-or-nothing types who enjoy contrast. Eating is more fun, after all, when hunger is extreme. There is even some evidence that the "gorging" impulse is a genetic holdover from our eat-it-while-you-can caveman days.

But for other people, people like Barbara, there's something a little more murky going on. Barbara looks to her one big meal a day not just as a pleasure, but as a tranquilizer, an antidote for stress. What Barbara fails to realize, however, is that by eating just one meal a day she is adding to the very stress she's trying to combat. Her blood sugar drops drastically as a result of her meal-skipping, which makes her irritable and hence much more sensitive to the pressures of her job and family alike. By 5:00 P.M. she's as testy as a rattlesnake—just ask her children, who sometimes get in her way as she's making dinner.

But it "all feels worth it" once Barbara can sit down to her roast beef and gravy. So the pattern—and the 20 unwanted pounds—roll on.

Why can't Barbara's exercise program turn things around?

Barbara participates in a company-sponsored aerobics class during her lunch break at work three days a week, but because she does that on an empty stomach, too, she hates it even more than she would otherwise. This leaves her feeling even grumpier by the time she gets home, so she's likely to go for three scoops of gravy on her roast beef instead of two, and maybe some extra chocolate ice cream because she's "earned it."

It's a nasty pattern that people like Barbara get themselves into. The more Barbara feels stressed, the more she eats. And the more she eats, the more she feels she must _not_ eat the next day, which only makes her feel more stressed. The solution, of course, is simply for Barbara to eat smaller meals more frequently—something we'll be looking at in greater detail later. First, however, a word on the types of food Barbara eats. They're a weight loser's Waterloo.

Type

Even though Barbara's total caloric intake for an average day is not out of line for someone of her weight and activity level, she remains 20 pounds "plump." Where's the hitch?

The hitch is that Barbara's diet is high in sugar and fat, the combination of which treats fat cells to a smorgasbord. Sugar calls up insulin, and one of the effects of insulin is to encourage calories to be stored as fat rather than burned for energy. What's worse, the combination of a high-sugar and high-fat diet may add up to more than the sum of its parts. According to studies conducted on rats by Lawrence Oscai and colleagues from the University of Illinois at Chicago, "Apparently, sugar and fat together in the diet have a mild additive effect on body fat content." The researchers found a 5 percent increase in body fat when sugar was added to a high-fat diet, even though no extra calories were consumed.

So what happens when the insulin in Barbara's bloodstream, which has been called up by the sheer size of her meal in addition to the sugar in her soft drink and chocolate ice cream, meets up with the fat from her roast beef and gravy?

Fat cells get a feast. Insulin makes them hypersensitive for storage, and dietary fat comes along to give them all the wrong thing to store. At 9 calories per gram as opposed to 4 for carbohydrates and protein, fat makes tough baggage to get rid of once tucked away.

But the drawbacks of a high-fat diet don't stop there. We've said this before, but it bears repeating: Because dietary fat is very similar to body fat in the first place, it requires very little biochemical energy to become body fat. Only about 3 calories for every 100 calories consumed are required for the conversion process. Carbohydrates, by contrast, require 23 percent of the available energy, and because the conversion of carbohydrates to fat is so costly and inefficient, the body hates to do it. This could work to Barbara's advantage if she would just switch to a low-fat, high–complex carbohydrate diet. Even if she consumed the same number of calories, she could lose weight. Here's how.

To avoid conversion, the body will increase its ability to store carbohydrate as glycogen, but that doesn't go very far. The next step is an increase in metabolic rate in an attempt to burn off the extra carbohydrate instead of converting it to fat. In addition, the Thermic Effect of Food (TEF)—the energy cost associated with digestion and absorption—climbs to a higher level for carbohydrates. Add a walk immediately after eating, and the TEF shoots even higher. These adaptations are great, and Barbara could be burning off excess calories effortlessly, simply because she replaced dietary fat with complex carbohydrates. What's more, because fat contains 9 calories per gram compared to carbohydrate's 4, Barbara could eat more food than before but take in fewer calories.

It's no longer a surprise to nutritionists that a diet high in fat is much more apt to put on weight than a diet equal in calories but lower in fat. The biochemical chain of events created by a high-fat diet can be difficult for even the most vigorous of exercise programs to reverse. If you're a fan of fast food and you also belong to a fitness club, you've probably learned this first hand. Sweat does a poor job of melting the grease. Stay tuned for more on the diet/body fat connection.

22

Lipo-Fitness to the Rescue

Stamford

Tell me what you eat, and I will tell you what you are.
—Anthelm Brillat-Savarin, 1755–1826

I must confess that when Porter came to me with *Fitness Without Exercise* as the title for this book, I had my reservations. I know you're supposed to come up with catchy titles in this book business, but catchy in the way that quicksand is catchy? Would we really be suggesting that superior health could be achieved without any attention being paid to aerobic exercise? That heart disease could be avoided, that strokes could be avoided, that obesity and diabetes and high blood pressure could be avoided? Exercise scientists like myself had worked for twenty years to show how aerobic exercise combats these "afflictions of modern living." Was I really willing to contest these findings and put my hard-earned reputation on the line in the process?

The more closely I looked at the evidence–and myself as living proof of that evidence—the more I became convinced that our title was not an unfair exaggeration at all. It was such a bold statement of the truth that it only *sounded* like quackery. It saw through twenty years of hazy uncertainty with such brightness and vision that it had blinded me at first.

But I have grown used to the light. I can now see where we have gone wrong and where we need to go from here to go right. We need to put the aerobic era behind us. The era inspired great science, science that has been invaluable in helping us to understand the causes of heart attack, stroke, diabetes, high blood pressure, and obesity. Where the movement stumbled, however, was in offering itself as the best *cure* for these disorders. Yes, aerobic exercise can reduce risk factors for all of the "diseases of civilization" mentioned, but only indirectly at best, and only with considerable investments of both effort and time. We need to thank the aerobic crusade for its help, but we need now to move on to what can be far more effective in accomplishing the goals the crusade had set out to achieve.

The time has come for a fresh start, a new approach—one that will fulfill expectations created by the aerobics movement. We offer lipo-fitness as the solution. "Lipo" is the medical term for fat, and the lipo-fitness approach entails reducing dietary fat—and saturated fat especially—to minimal levels. In conjunction with moderate day-to-day physical activity to increase caloric expenditure and to maintain muscle tone, joint flexibility, and bone strength, the lipo-fitness lifestyle delivers the health benefits that aerobics promised twenty years ago. But to accomplish this, we must move the battle from the gymnasium to the kitchen.

Go ahead, open your refrigerator door. If you're like most Americans, you'll see the real enemy staring you square in the face. Lack of exercise hasn't been the major factor responsible for 500,000 American heart attacks every year—butter, mayonnaise, and salami are much more culpable. The past twenty years have seen us trying to fix *from the outside*, with exercise, problems that have been arising *from the inside* due to our high-fat diets. We've been like bozo mechanics trying to do tune-ups on engines that haven't been running right simply because we've been trying to operate them on bad gas.

And sorry, salami fans, but "bad gas" has been what we've been fueling up on since the Industrial Revolution brought us prosperity and the tabletop assassin we have come to know and love as saturated fat. As the saturated fat content of the typical American diet has risen since the early 1900s, so have rates of heart disease. Only in the past few years have enough Americans wised up to the connection to begin to reverse the trend, but we still have miles to go before bringing the fat content of the average American diet to within healthful levels. We currently get about 40 percent of our calories from fat when we *should* be getting only about 20 percent. (The American Heart Association says 30 percent, but they've been regrettably conservative in responding to the writing on artery walls.) Fat in the diet becomes fat in the blood, which becomes material for arterial plaque. Had the aerobics movement made that better known twenty years ago, we might not be doing tens of thousands of coronary bypass surgeries every year in the United States today—more than a few of them on joggers.

The "Blast Furnace" Fallacy

But no, ask the average exercise buff why he or she works out and one of the reasons is apt to be "Because it lets me eat more of the foods I love."

Is that reasonable logic? Can a 500-calorie workout pardon the nutritional crimes of a 500-calorie hot fudge sundae? Can the wafer-thin triathelete who trains for three hours a day fuel himself on anything he darned well pleases?

One way to answer that is to reveal a little-known biological fact: Ninety percent of the cells that presently make up your body were not with you as recently as a few months ago. You have a new heart, new lungs, new muscles, new eyeballs. Even most of your bones are new. Only nerve cells have a lifespan longer than a few months. The rest of you expires and needs to be replaced constantly.

And where does the raw material for all this cellular reconstruction come from?

No, not from a lifetime membership to Fitness America. It comes from the food you eat. We tend to think of food just as fuel, but it's much more than that. It's the biological bricks and mortar of which we're made, and if the bricks and mortar are defective, *we're* going to be defective. Good genes can intervene somewhat, like a clever architect, but even the best of genes cannot build a temple from Twinkies.

A cute but oversimplified analogy?

Consider this: Research gathered by the U.S. Department of Health indicates that as many as two-thirds of all causes of death in this country are in some way diet-related. Heart disease, cancer, diabetes, high blood pressure, and strokes—all are cordially invited by our less-than-optimal diets.

Think about that. Food is supposed to sustain life, and nearly a third of the world's population still does not have enough, but in America food *threatens* life. I passed a billboard recently that said, "Beat the Burger Blahs, Try a Steak Sandwich at So and So's."

Wow! We've grown accustomed to feeding ourselves so excessively in this country that even those two all-beef patties dripping with gourmet sauce are losing their appeal. Where did we go wrong?

It could be argued that our gluttony is an inevitable result of our affluence—the Romans, after all, were no Pritikins—but the Japanese are certainly no paupers, and they boast one of the healthiest diets and lowest rates of heart disease in the world. Besides, it doesn't take being a Rockefeller to dine at McDonald's. I should know. I did it every day for lunch for several years—two cheeseburgers with extra pickles, a large order of fries, a carton of whole milk, and a cherry pie. I became such a regular that the girl behind the counter would begin pleading my case for extra pickles to the grill-boy the moment she saw me walk in.

How could I, an exercise physiologist and health "expert," justify a diet like that?

In all honesty, I never stopped to think at the time that I was doing anything wrong. My McDonald's years were during the late seventies and early eighties, before the dangers of dietary fat captured the attention of health professionals. Besides, my scientific efforts were devoted to improving physical performance. Health promotion was of little concern, especially since I assumed that I was already at the top of the heap, believing like other exercise buffs that my fitness was protecting me. I was convinced that my grueling daily workouts had my body running like a blast furnace capable of totally obliterating anything I put into it. My diet wasn't adding fat to the outside of my body, after all, so why should I fear a buildup of fat anywhere inside? I had the endurance of a sled dog and—with the exception of a stubborn set of love handles—a physique as padded as a park bench. Shouldn't it follow that my arteries and blood would be as fat-free as the rest of me?

The answer to that came as quite a shock when I had my cholesterol tested. It was 210 mg./dl.—not dangerously high but certainly higher than I would have expected for a guy with a workout schedule like mine. Worse yet, my all-important HDL level—the "good" cholesterol that helps keep arteries clean—was a measly 34 mg./dl. A man my age, even a sedentary man, should have a level in the low to mid 40s. These numbers gave me a very disturbing total cholesterol-to-HDL ratio of 6.2 to 1.

My reaction to these figures?

It was a laughable one now that I look back on it: I doubled my running mileage. It didn't even occur to me to clean up my diet. I felt I had to burn that cholesterol out of my blood with exercise, so I hit the roads with a vengeance. Six months later I had my cholesterol checked again, fully expecting to see a dramatic drop.

But I got not even a droop—no change at all despite six grueling months. Not even an improvement in my HDLs. It was then that I began to question exercise as the great junk food incinerator. And it scared me. Would I have to change my junk food ways? Pack a tuna sandwich to replace my beloved lunch beneath the golden arches? Eat oatmeal for breakfast instead of bacon and eggs? Sit down to broiled fish for dinner instead of Polish sausage?

As a scientist and as someone concerned about his health, I had to give it a try. I made changes gradually—and not easily—but to make a long story short, they worked. My total cholesterol dropped 40 points in six months, and mostly just from eating a healthier lunch.

Then I married Joy. My eating habits had much improved by that time, but they still left lots of room for improvement. Compared to Joy's standards, in fact, you could say that I was still eating like William "The Refrigerator" Perry.

At first Joy surrendered to pressure and cooked sludge for me and my two teenage sons, but eventually she convinced us at least to try a better way. We started eating more complex carbohydrates—in the form of rice, pasta, potatoes, and beans—and broiled chicken and fish replaced hamburgers, hot dogs, and fatty steaks. Oatmeal and fresh fruit replaced bacon and eggs for breakfast, and snacking got done on the likes of popcorn, vegetable sticks, and homemade bread rather than ice cream, cookies, and potato chips.

The results were stunning. Within about six months my cholesterol was into the 140s and eventually dropped to its current level of 101 mg.dl. Joy enjoys a cholesterol level of about 140.

But don't we feel deprived eating so healthfully?

That's been the best news of all. I've never enjoyed eating more in my life. Nor have I ever eaten *as much* in my life. By reducing the fat in our diets, we've reduced a good deal of the calories and hence been able to increase the amount we eat in terms of sheer bulk. This doesn't mean we're nutritionally perfect, however. We follow what we call the "80/20 Rule," eating healthfully most of the time but splurging without guilt when we go to parties or dine out. And when the mood strikes, there's an occasional pizza, ice cream treat, or devilish dessert at home.

We'll be talking more about the dietary control of serum cholesterol later, and we'll provide specific recipes for some of the meals Joy and I eat, but for the time being let it be said again that *the best way to keep fat out of your blood and your arteries is not to put it in your mouth in the first place.* My own experience and Joy's proved it, and controlled scientific studies also have shown it. Several cases of sudden death among dedicated joggers with high cholesterol levels—some in excess of 300 mg.dl.—have been reported, and it's not unusual for Olympic-caliber endurance athletes to demonstrate cholesterol levels of 240 mg./dl. or more. Other research has shown that vegetarians have lower cholesterol levels, and thus a lower risk of heart disease, than meat-eating marathoners.

Diet matters more than exercise in the prevention of coronary artery disease—I'm convinced of that now. Thinking that a heavy workout schedule can nullify the effects of a fatty diet is like thinking you can get rid of the effects of using cheap gas by driving your car fast. A high-performance engine needs the best and cleanest-burning fuel possible.

Fat Sticks to the Ribs As Well As to the Arteries

But my cholesterol levels aside, something else happened when I reduced the fat in my diet, and it may be of even more interest to a lot of you than my improved odds against heart disease: I lost body fat. For years, no matter how hard I worked out, I carried a pair of not-so-adorable "love handles"—deposits of fat at my sides just above the beltline. They would jiggle as I jogged, and they drove me nuts. I resorted to high-waisted shorts—you know the type, and now you know why men wear them.

Well, with the advent of my lipo-fitness lifestyle and the end of my high-fat diet, the love handles started dwindling. Without doing any additional exercise—actually doing less—I lost a good portion of those grips that had been with me since I had bulked-up for power lifting in my twenties.

The disappearance surprised me at the time, but research done since then has made the vanishing act very understandable. Fat, you see, is more fattening—calorie for calorie—than carbohydrate or protein, and not just because it contains more calories per gram. If you ate 300 calories in the form of fat, those 300 calories would be more likely to "stick to your ribs" than 300 calories from carbohydrate or protein. Witness results of a research study that demonstrated that middle-aged men overfed a diet high in fat gained 30 pounds in just three months while another group fed *even more calories* in the form of carbohydrate took an average of *seven* months to gain 30 pounds.

Not only are you likely to gain fat, but the fat you gain from eating fat is likely to be in the abdomen.

Why?

Possibly because fat is digested by the liver, which is located in the abdominal area. The digested fat may linger before heading out to other areas of the body—if, in fact, it ever heads out at all. The unique preference for converting dietary fat to abdominal fat has been demonstrated in rats, but there's reason to believe similar mechanisms are at work in humans. But more on this in our chapter on the "Humpty Dumpty Syndrome."

Dietary fat is at the bottom of most of our weight problems as well as cardiovascular problems in this country, and the sooner we realize that, the better off our hearts as well as our physiques are going to be. The cellulite, saddle bags, potbellies, and spare tires leave little doubt that the fitness movement's not working. It's time for a change. Lipo-fitness will succeed where aerobic fitness has failed.

Read on.

23

The Humpty Dumpty Syndrome: Heart Hazard Number One?

Stamford

I look upon it, that he who does not mind his belly will hardly mind anything else.
—Samuel Johnson, 1709–1784

No doubt you've seen it and maybe you're even guilty of it: that full-bellied look, narrow at the hips but W-I-D-E at the waist. Legs and arms can actually be quite lean, but get in around the equator and things get big in a hurry.

What's responsible for the "I swallowed a watermelon" look? And more importantly, what does it mean for the heart?

Research is showing that abdominal obesity may be a seriously underrated hazard, a condition far more dangerous than higher levels of obesity that are more evenly distributed. Least dangerous of all appears to be the predominantly female pattern of fat being carried in the area of the hips, buttocks, and thighs.

137

And yet, where have most exercise programs focused their fat-loss promises?

On the hips, buttocks, and thighs. It's yet another example of how the fitness effort has missed a crucial point. Thighs, even if they're thunderous, aren't killing 500,000 Americans every year of heart disease. The blame goes to abdominal girth. Take Ed, for example, a man in his late forties who came to me for advice on what to do about a cholesterol level of 310. He was interested mainly in improving his fitness, but when I saw his stomach I suggested we make weight loss his primary goal.

"I don't need to lose weight, Dr. Stamford, this is just the way I'm built. Here, feel this thing. I know it's big, but it's as hard as a rock. See, there's not an ounce of fat on it," he said as I gave him the poke he asked for. "Where's the weight loss going to come from?"

There was no arguing that Ed's stomach was indeed firm. But that didn't mean it wasn't fat. It was time for an anatomy lesson. I told Ed that the only reason his stomach was firm was because the fat responsible for it was located beneath his abdominal muscles rather than on top of them. His stomach muscles were stretched tighter than a banjo string trying to hold the fat in place, and that's why his stomach appeared so hard.

But Ed wouldn't buy it. No, his wife was the one who needed to lose weight, he told me. She was the one, after all, whose thighs jiggled so much "it was a crime."

"To the eye maybe, Ed, but not to the heart," I told him. "Your wife's thighs do not pose a fraction of the coronary risks that your potbelly does. What is your diet like?"

When Ed went on to describe the ham and eggs for breakfast and predominantly fast foods after that, I wasn't surprised. As you'll recall from the previous chapter, dietary fat, in addition to being more fattening than carbohydrates and protein from the standpoint of caloric density, has a far greater tendency to result in fat accumulation in the abdominal area.

"Ed, your diet is feeding that thing," I told him. "Even if you ate the same number of calories, you would see some shrinkage if you ate less fat."

I went so far as to tell Ed my own story of the vanishing love handles when I stopped lunching at McDonald's and cut out other sources of fat, but he still seemed skeptical. He was convinced that because his stomach was "hard," he was not fat. And because his wife's thighs were "soft," she was. It's a mistake that's been plaguing our understanding of obesity, and hence our success at dealing with it, since the invention of the steam bath. Let's take an inside look at why fat in the area of the abdomen, far more than fat anywhere else on the body, is the true culprit in the heart disease process.

Fat Too Close for Comfort

All body fat releases fat molecules into the bloodstream, but the location of the body fat is important because it dictates how many of those molecules will eventually get to the liver, and hence spur that organ to increase its output of LDL cholesterol, the bad kind suspected of accumulating on artery walls. The farther from the liver the fat is located, the better, because fat molecules have to travel a considerable distance through the bloodstream before the liver is reached. This increases the likelihood that the molecules will be picked up by muscle cells on some other type of tissue and be put to a legitimate use. The result is that relatively few of the fat molecules are apt to converge on the liver at any one time, thus minimizing the danger that the liver will be forced into an inordinately high LDL output. Fat located far from the liver (in the areas of the hips, thighs, arms, and back, for example) is thought to pose relatively little cardiovascular risk for this reason.

Not so, however, with fat located around the abdomen, and especially fat located *beneath* the abdominal muscles. When fat molecules enter the blood from intra-abdominal fat like Ed's, they go to the liver directly by way of the hepatic portal vein, the result being a barrage on the liver that can cause it to increase its output of LDL cholesterol dramatically. The danger of such an increase, of course, is that these LDLs will remain true to their reputation of contributing the buildup of plaque on artery walls.

But location is only half the problem of abdominal fat. Compared to fat located elsewhere on the body, intra-abdominal fat—Ed's kind, which actually surrounds the trunk's internal organs—is metabolically hyperactive. Scientists have compared intra-abdominal fat to fat from other parts of the body and found that it behaves very differently. Whereas most fat needs considerable coaxing from hormones such as adrenaline to enter the bloodstream, intra-abdominal fat (called visceral fat) needs no such hormonal help. Worse yet, if a fat-mobilizing hormone such as adrenaline does enter the picture, visceral fat goes crazy, entering the bloodstream in a veritable torrent. The danger of this, of course, is that the liver gets flooded worse than ever, and the arteries ultimately pay the price. Researchers speculate that this may be why emotional stress, which is an adrenaline stimulator, may be such a heart disease threat. Marry emotional stress with a big stomach and you've got jeopardy times two.

But back to Ed. When I got through explaining all this to him, he finally seemed to understand. He even had a good question: "What if someone has a big stomach that's not hard, but flabby? Does that mean he's not in as much trouble because his fat is on the outside of his stomach muscles, where it can't be so bothersome to the liver?"

"You mean someone like Santa Claus, Ed, whose stomach shakes like a bowlful of jelly?"

I went on to explain that someone like Santa is in double trouble. A large and protruding stomach that's also flabby means that fat tissue probably has filled up all available space inside the abdominal cavity, thus needing to spill over to the outside. This degree of obesity can pose blood pressure problems in addition to making even worse the cholesterol complications caused by excessive fat inside the abdomen. Add the diabetic risks and back problems posed by Santa's kind of obesity, and it's no wonder the man works only one day a year.

The Tale of the Tape

Now that I had Ed believing, I asked him if he'd be willing to undergo some diagnostic measurement. He said he would, so we measured his waist to the nearest quarter of an inch precisely at the level of his navel as he stood barechested and breathing normally. He came to 40 1/2 inches. Next we measured his hips, slightly lower down, precisely at the level of the hip bone. He came to 36 3/4 inches. We converted both figures to decimals (40.5 and 36.75), divided the waist measurement by the hip measurement (40.5 ÷ 36.75), and got 1.1 after rounding to the nearest tenth.

It wasn't a good number. According to research done in at least three large-scale studies, Ed's waist-to-hip ratio (WHR) put him in about the top 5 percent of all men tested. A man should have a ratio of closer to 0.9, and preferably about 0.85. Recommended levels for women are even lower—between about 0.7 and 0.8. Ed wanted to know the implications of his high number.

"Research is showing that a high waist-to-hip ratio indicates increased risks not just of heart disease, but of diabetes and strokes as well," I told him.

And indeed, Ed's cholesterol level of 310 was proof that his Humpty Dumpty profile already was heading him for some sort of cardiovascular fall. I told Ed he needed to make drastic reductions in his intake of dietary fat and that he needed to be more active as well.

He wasn't happy, so I thought the least I could do was rally him with the one bit of good news research has discovered regarding the all-important WHR measurement: "Fat in the area of the abdomen is more easily lost than fat elsewhere on the body," I told him.

Men in one study lost nearly twice as much fat from their abdominal areas as from other areas of the body when they dramatically increased their activity levels. The reason abdominal fat gets lost more easily, the researchers speculated, is that the same metabolic hyperactivity that gets it in trouble with the liver also makes it more available as an energy source: It's readily available in the blood, so it's readily available for use.

When I explained to Ed that this, unfortunately, was the reason so many women find fat in the area of the hips and thighs to be relatively resistant to weight loss, he became suddenly sympathetic. He told me that his wife had been trying to lose weight from her hips and thighs ever since he could remember, but to no avail.

There's a trade-off being made here, though, I had to tell him. Yes, the female tendency to carry fat in the area of the hips and thighs may make fat loss more difficult for women, but it also tends to protect them from the heart disease and diabetic dangers that abdominal fat imposes. Studies show that women can carry from 40 to 60 pounds more fat than men, if they carry it in the hips, thighs, and upper arms, without suffering from undue cardiovascular risks. Women who tend to carry their fat in the area of the stomach as men do, however, lose this protective edge.

It's certainly something to keep in mind as you evaluate your own weight-loss needs. If you're carrying your excess weight low, as a pear, more than around the middle, as an egg, rest assured that you are not at equal risk for the kind of cardiovascular crash that faces Humpty Dumpty types like Ed. This may seem like a small consolation, but it's not. The cosmetic drawbacks of large thighs should be considered tiny compared to the life-threatening burdens of a heart attack or stroke.

And note, too, that the best way of losing fat, no matter where it is, is to eat less fat and to increase physical activity. Any exercise program that promises "spot reduction" is pulling more than just your leg. People in a 1984 study published in the *Research Quarterly for Exercise and Sport* failed to reduce abdominal obesity at all despite a twenty-seven-day training regimen that included an average of 185 sit-ups a day.

Their efforts would have been better spent, as we hope to convince you before this book is through, by reducing the fat in their diets and playing badminton or walking the dog.

24

Fiendish Fat, a Closer Look

Shimer

Fattenin' hogs ain't in luck.
—Joel Chandler Harris, 1848–1908

If you were given the job of concocting a food component hazardous to human health, you would be hard pressed to come up with something more insidious than saturated fat.

And yet there it is, making up over half of all the fat we consume, making our mouths water in hamburgers, hot dogs, milk, cheese, ice cream, potato chips, and even apple pie. The foods that have grown the dearest to our hearts are the most dangerous for our hearts. You couldn't have written a worse script if you had tried.

An exaggeration? A red flag when something in a soft pink might more accurately represent the truth?

Unfortunately not. Too much fat in our diets—and saturated fat especially—currently stands accused of being a contributor either directly or indirectly to heart attacks, strokes, high blood pressure, diabetes, obesity, and cancers of the colon, prostate, uterus, and breast. Next to cigarette smoking, excess dietary fat bears the burden of being the single most preventable cause of death that we face. It's not a very flattering scenario for a nation that prides itself on being on a health kick.

How has it happened? Where has all the fat come from? And how can we most effectively avoid the "grease spill" that threatens our internal environments?

First, let's understand the enemy.

Not all fat is bad. Some is healthful and necessary, in fact. Fat helps distribute and store the fat-soluble vitamins A, D, E, and K; it keeps skin adequately lubricated and contributes to the production of essential compounds called prostaglandins, which exert control over many of the body's important biochemical activities.

But here's the catch: The amount of fat needed to perform these essential activities is less than one-twelfth of the amount most Americans currently consume. A diet that derives only 3 percent of its calories from fat would be sufficient for carrying out fat's vital functions, and yet most of us get about 40 percent of our calories from fat, saturated and unsaturated. What's more—and here's where the typical American diet really shows its lunacy—the type of fat needed to meet the body's needs is of the unsaturated variety. Saturated fat serves virtually no useful biological function whatsoever, and yet most of us consume more than twice as much of it as unsaturated fat.

Beginning to get a feel for the burdens that saturated fat imposes? Here's a food component that's not just useless, but proven harmful, and it's making up a whopping two-thirds of our fat intake and nearly 30 percent of the calories of the average American diet.

A Chemistry Lesson

But how can one form of fat differ so greatly from another? And to what does the term "saturated" actually refer?

Saturated fat occurs primarily in animal foods—meats, eggs, milk, butter, and cheese—and it differs from unsaturated fat in a very fundamental way. All fats—whether saturated, monounsaturated, or polyunsaturated—are made up of strings of carbon atoms with hydrogen atoms attached, but that's where the similarity ends. In a polyunsaturated fat, two or more of the carbon atoms do not have hydrogen atoms attached, while in a monounsaturated fat only one of the carbon atoms is left vacant. But in a saturated fat, you've got a hydrogen "full house." All of the carbon atoms have hydrogen partners, so the fat is said to be "saturated" with hydrogen.

This may sound like a lot of chemical mumbo-jumbo, but as far as the liver is concerned the difference is very real. Research leaves no doubt that a diet high in saturated fat can cause the liver to increase its output of cholesterol, and LDL cholesterol especially, the kind most prone to contribute to arterial clogging. Worse yet, saturated fat in the blood can increase the stickiness of blood platelets, the blood cells that can form clots leading to heart attacks and strokes. Add the tendency of saturated fat to raise blood pressure and you've got triple trouble.

But saturated fat is capable of fouling up more than just the circulatory system, unfortunately. Studies show it can increase risks of diabetes, gall bladder disease, and cancers of the colon, prostate, uterus, and breast. It's not friendly stuff, or at least not in the quantities we are presently asking our bodies to deal with. Not until the livestock industry started fattening up our meat sources did we have to contend with much saturated fat at all, in fact. We had milk, butter, and cheese, of course, but even those sources of saturated fat are relatively recent, given the 250,000-year history of the human digestive system as we currently know it. The way our bodies handle food has changed precious little since prehistoric times, and yet the foods we now eat have changed quite dramatically. Anthropologists estimate that our intake of saturated fat has increased since prehistoric times by as much as sixfold, from less than 5 percent of calories to our current 30 percent. No wonder our arterial plumbing has been needing so much service from bypass surgery and angioplasty lately. We've been trying to pump too much "sludge."

No Help from Exercise

Worse yet, the exercise movement has been giving us the impression for the past twenty years that we could run away from the dangers of saturated fat. That fallacy, combined with the increasing prevalence of saturated fat in our foods, has proven to be a very unhealthy combination. The Centers for Disease Control (CDC) in Atlanta reported in April of 1989 that while deaths from heart disease have declined by about 20 percent in the past twenty years, the number of people hospitalized for heart disease has *risen* by about 30 percent. Seven hundred and eighty-four men per 100,000 were hospitalized for heart disease in 1970, but by 1986 the figure had climbed to 1,066. The rate for women jumped from 570 to 718 per 100,000.

Is that simply evidence of better heart disease detection?

Perhaps, but it also suggests greater heart disease prevalence. Deaths from heart disease have declined because doctors have gotten better at keeping clogged arteries from being fatal, but we, unfortunately, also have gotten better at clogging our arteries in the first place. Most recent surveys suggest that as many as 60 million adults in the United States have cholesterol levels that put them at a substantial heart disease risk.

The era of "lipo-fitness" may soon be upon us, however, as the U.S. Surgeon General's *Report on Nutrition and Health* in July of 1988 finally declared war on fat as war had been declared on smoking fifteen years earlier. "Dietary changes can improve the health of Americans, and the primary dietary priority is reduced consumption of fat, especially saturated fat," stated the report. The battle line—finally—appears to have been drawn by the federal government itself.

Those Other Fats Aren't All Friendly, Either

But if saturated fat is such a demon, can other fats really be so kind? The polyunsaturated and monounsaturated fats that are being presented as so beneficial in magazine ads and on TV?

Studies suggest that replacing saturated fat in the diet with unsaturated fat may indeed help to lower serum cholesterol, but this should not be interpreted to mean that unsaturated fat may be consumed in large quantities. The American Heart Association wants no more than 30 percent of our calories coming from fat regardless of what type the fat is, and many authorities, ourselves included, are calling for even less fat than that—about 20 percent of calories.

Why?

Because all fats, regardless of type, contain the same whopping 9 calories per gram and hence are a major instigator of obesity. What's more, although some researchers claim that unsaturated fats lower cholesterol levels, the reasons are not clear. Substituting unsaturated fat for saturated fat may lower cholesterol simply because the substitution results in less saturated fat being consumed. There's not a lipid researcher anywhere who would advise adding unsaturated fat to a diet already high in saturated fat as a way of lowering serum cholesterol. Your goal should be to reduce your intake of *all* types of fat, while working to see that the fats you do get are primarily of the polyunsaturated and monounsaturated variety. Ideally, the calories you get from saturated fat should comprise no more than about 10 percent of your overall caloric intake, with less being even better. This allows the other 10 to 20 percent of your fat calories (depending on whether you're going for a 20 percent or a 30 percent total fat limit) to come from the more healthful polyunsaturated and monounsaturated varieties.

But how can the difference of a few hydrogen atoms make unsaturated fat friendly and saturated fat downright dangerous?

Researchers aren't totally sure yet. The difference appears to lie in how the different types of fat are metabolized by the liver. Scientists do know this, however. Unlike the other fats, saturated fat is a primary material from which cholesterol is made. The liver manufactures between 80 and 90 percent of all the cholesterol in your body, and saturated fat is one

of the major sources the liver uses. Strange as it may seem, eating cholesterol directly in foods such as shellfish, organ meats, and eggs appears
to have less of a cholesterol-raising effect than eating foods high in saturated fat. The reason may be that the body senses a need to cut back on
cholesterol production when it finds itself confronted by excess cholesterol
in the diet directly. With too much saturated fat, on the other hand, the
body may not sense such an emergency and hence just continue on with
its cholesterol production.

   As proof of just what a cholesterol-raising scoundrel saturated fat can
be, research has shown that even if people were put on a diet that derived
only 25 percent of its calories from fat, they failed to see any drops in
cholesterol at all if the kind of fat they were restricted to was primary of
the saturated variety. When the same people were put on a low-fat diet
that derived its fat primarily from unsaturated fat, however, their cholesterol levels fell an average of 20 percent.

Finding and Avoiding the Enemy

Saturated fat is more than just unhealthy, however. It's sly. It can hide
in foods you may not think of as high-fat sources. Many people who avoid
red meat because of its saturated fat, for example, are surprised to learn
that a single ounce of most hard cheeses (cheddar, swiss, colby, muenster)
harbors more saturated fat than a 3.5-ounce serving of lean T-bone steak.
Or that there's saturated fat in the coconut oil in their bowl of "healthy"
granola. Or that a breaded fish fillet that's been deep-fried can serve up
more saturated fat than a hamburger. Baked goods, too, can hide a lot of
saturated fat, especially those of "gourmet" caliber, because butter, beef
lard, or a hydrogenated vegetable oil may be a prominent ingredient.

   And indeed, the blame for much of the unrecognized saturated fat in
our diet lies with the hydrogenation process. A fat that has been hydrogenated is one that has been made more saturated by a process that gives
hydrogen partners to some of those lonely carbon atoms we talked about.
It's done by blowing hydrogen gas through vats of unsaturated oil that
has been pressurized and heated. The reason it's done is to give foods
containing these fats added shelf life. Hydrogenated fats take longer than
unsaturated fats to turn "rancid," a process whereby a fat begins to spoil
due to prolonged exposure to oxygen. But like the salt that's used to help
preserve processed meats, what's good for the food is not always good for
the body. Hydrogenated vegetable oils, which have found their way into
everything from puddings to cookies to fried chicken, have been a major
contributor to the great American "grease spill" that presently engulfs us.

Add the recent invasion of the palm oils (coconut, palm, and palm kernel), which are highly saturated, and it's clear that we need to be on our toes to keep from being felled by the slick. The chart that concludes this chapter should help you.

A Word on Those Fish Fats

And what about the worth of the special type of polyunsaturated fat in fish that scientists call omega-3 fatty acids? Are omega-3s all they've been cracked up to be as defenders against heart disease? Should you be taking fish oil capsules? Should you be buying fresh flounder for twice as much per pound as you can buy chicken breasts?

Two answers to those questions:

1. Yes, the type of fat prevalent in cold-water fish has been shown in reputable studies to lower serum cholesterol and triglycerides as well as to reduce the tendency of the blood to clot—three important benefits for anyone trying to avoid both heart attack and stroke. But . . .
2. No, you don't have to cut into your lottery ticket budget to be able to afford fish oil capsules or swordfish for $7.00 a pound to get these heart-health omega 3s (also referred to as eicosapentanoic acid, or EPA). Canned tuna is an excellent source of omega-3s, as are sardines, canned mackerel, and salmon. Fish does not have to be fresh or costly to be abundant in EPA power.

Fish oil capsules?

You're better off getting your EPA from fish itself than from capsules, especially if you think the capsules can make up for a diet that's atrocious in other respects. Eating fish offers the opportunity to substitute unsaturated fat for saturated, and the lower saturated fat intake will lower your cholesterol. Also beware that fish oil capsules can be extremely high in cholesterol, and it's also possible to ingest toxic amounts of vitamins A and D with these supplements.

Where do chicken and turkey fit into a cholesterol-lowering game plan?

Properly prepared, they can be almost as heart-healthy as fish. They contain no EPA, but they are low in saturated fat—light-meat turkey especially. Cooking chicken and turkey with skin removed lowers fat content even more. Their meat might not taste as "juicy" when cooked skinless, but the sooner you teach your taste buds that juicy is synonymous with fatty, the healthier your heart will be. Fried chicken, which can serve up as much saturated fat as a hamburger, should be reserved for special occasions only.

Seven Fat-Fighting Strategies

The fat-fighting game can seem confusing, but it doesn't have to be. Here are some tips to help you:

1. *Try to restrict your fat intake to no more than 45 grams a day.* Assuming your total food intake comes to about 2,000 calories a day, this will assure that no more than 20 percent of these calories will be coming from fat.
2. *Try to restrict your intake of saturated fat to less than 15 grams a day.* This will allow the unsaturated fat in your diet to exceed the saturated fat by a very heart-healthy 2 to 1 margin.
3. *Try to eat fish at least twice a week.* Not only will this help to keep your total fat intake low, it will guarantee that you're getting healthful amounts of omega-3 fatty acids, which research has shown can control serum cholesterol and triglycerides and also reduce the tendency of the blood to clot, a major factor contributing to heart attacks and stroke.
4. *Try to limit cholesterol intake to less than 300 mg. a day.* Whether or not dietary cholesterol increases serum cholesterol significantly, research suggests that it's still a good idea to keep your intake low. (See the chart that follows for the greatest cholesterol offenders.)
5. *Use margarine instead of butter, but use it sparingly.* Soft-tub and liquid margarines are best because their fat tends to be the least saturated. Margarine still contains as many calories and as much fat (although unsaturated) as butter, however, so go easy.
6. *Choose polyunsaturated and monounsaturated oils for salads and cooking.* Good "polys" are corn, sunflower, safflower, and rapeseed (also called canola oil). Good "monos" (which new research suggests may be even more heart-healthy than polys because they lower LDL cholesterol without lowering HDLs) are olive, sesame, and peanut oil.
7. *And perhaps most important of all, learn the simple formula for calculating fat content.* Food labels give you "calories per serving" and "grams of fat per serving," but most have not gone the next step and given us what we really need to know—"percent of calories from fat." You can determine fat percentages, however, simply by doing the following calculation:

- Multiply the "grams of fat per serving" by 9 (the number of calories in a single gram of fat).
- Divide this number by the "number of calories per serving" and multiply by 100 to get a percentage. For example:

> Milk (1 cup) contains 8 grams of fat and 150 calories
> 8 grams × 9 cals = 72 calories from fat
> 72 ÷ 150 = .48 × 100 = 48% fat

A Guide to the Greatest Fat Villains

The following foods are those you will need to avoid most to escape the hazards of saturated fat. Your goal, remember, should be to take in no more than about 45 grams of total fat, and no more than about 15 grams of saturated fat daily. Cholesterol should be limited to about 300 mg.

MEATS (3½ ounces cooked)	Cal.	% Fat	Total fat (gm.)	Sat. fat (gm.)	Choles. (mg.)
Ground beef, regular	274	66	20.1	7.3	84
Salami (3–4 slices)	262	71	20.7	9.0	65
Sausage (2)	312	78	27.0	11.4	67
Bologna (3–4 slices)	312	82	28.4	12.1	58
Bratwurst	301	77	25.7	9.3	60
Bacon	576	78	49.9	17.4	85
Corned beef, brisket	251	68	18.9	6.3	98
Spareribs, lean	397	69	30.4	11.8	121
Frankfurter, beef (2)	315	82	28.7	12.0	61
Frankfurter, turkey (2)	226	70	17.6	5.9	107
Frankfurter, chicken (2)	257	68	19.4	5.5	101
Bologna, turkey (3–4 slices)	199	69	15.3	5.1	99
Short ribs, lean	238	52	13.7	5.8	79

Fat content will vary somewhat in bologna, salami, and sausage, depending upon whether beef or pork is used.

DAIRY	Cal.	% Fat	Total fat (gm.)	Sat. fat (gm.)	Choles. (mg.)
Milk, whole (1 cup)	150	48	8.0	5.1	33
Sour cream (1 oz.)	61	87	5.9	3.7	12
Egg, chicken (whole)	79	64	5.6	1.7	274
Egg, chicken (yolk)	63	80	5.6	1.7	272
Butter, pat (1 tsp.)	34	100	3.8	2.5	11

CHEESES (1 ounce)	Cal.	% Fat	Total fat (gm.)	Sat. fat (gm.)	Choles. (mg.)
American	82	66	6.0	3.8	16
Feta	75	72	6.3	4.2	22

CHEESES (1 ounce)	Cal.	% Fat	Total fat (gm.)	Sat. fat (gm.)	Choles. (mg.)
Provolone	100	68	7.6	4.8	20
Limburger	93	75	7.8	4.8	26
Romano	110	63	8.4	4.9	29
Gouda	101	69	7.7	5.0	32
Swiss	107	65	7.7	5.0	26
Edam	101	70	7.8	5.0	25
Brick	105	72	8.4	5.3	27
Blue	100	73	8.1	5.3	21
Muenster	104	74	8.6	5.4	27
Parmesan	129	59	8.5	5.4	22
Monterey Jack	106	73	8.6	5.5	25
Roquefort	105	75	8.8	5.5	26
Colby	112	73	9.1	5.7	27
Cheddar	114	74	9.4	6.0	30
Ricotta, whole milk (4 oz.)	197	67	14.7	9.4	58
Cream cheese	99	90	9.9	6.2	31
Quiche Lorraine (⅛ 8″ pie)	600	72	48.0	23.2	285

SAUCES AND SALAD DRESSINGS	Cal.	% Fat	Total fat (gm.)	Sat. fat (gm.)	Choles. (mg.)
Hollandaise (½ cup)	353	87	34.1	20.9	94
Bearnaise (½ cup)	351	88	34.3	20.9	99
Mayonnaise (1 Tbsp.)	99	100	11.0	1.6	8
Thousand Island (1 Tbsp.)	59	86	5.6	.9	0
Italian (1 Tbsp.)	69	93	7.1	1.0	0
Russian (1 Tbsp.)	76	92	7.8	1.1	0
French (1 Tbsp.)	67	86	6.4	1.5	0
Blue cheese (1 Tbsp.)	77	93	7.9	1.5	0

NUTS AND SEEDS (1 ounce)	Cal.	% Fat	Total fat (gm.)	Sat. fat (gm.)	Choles. (mg.)
Hazelnuts	179	89	17.7	1.3	0
Almonds	167	80	14.8	1.4	0
Pecans	187	89	18.5	1.5	0
Sunflower seeds	165	77	14.1	1.5	0
Walnuts	182	87	17.6	1.6	0
Pistachios	164	75	13.7	1.7	0
Peanuts	164	76	13.8	1.9	0
Hickory nuts	187	88	18.3	2.0	0
Pumpkin seeds	148	73	12.0	2.3	0
Cashews	163	73	13.2	2.6	0
Macadamia nuts	199	95	21.0	3.1	0
Brazil nuts	186	91	18.8	4.6	0
Coconut meat	187	88	18.3	16.3	0

SNACKS AND MISCELLANEOUS	Cal.	% Fat	Total fat (gm.)	Sat. fat (gm.)	Choles. (mg.)
Milk chocolate (1 oz.)	145	56	9.0	5.4	6
Doughnut, cake (1)	210	51	11.9	2.8	20

SNACKS AND MISCELLANEOUS	Cal.	% Fat	Total fat (gm.)	Sat. fat (gm.)	Choles. (mg.)
Doughnut, glazed (1)	235	50	13.0	5.2	21
Peanut butter (1 Tbsp.)	95	77	8.1	1.4	0
Potato salad (1 cup)	358	52	20.7	3.6	170
Potato chips (1 oz.)	147	62	10.1	2.6	0
Corn chips (1 oz.)	155	52	8.9	1.4	25
Chocolate chip cookies (4)	185	54	11.1	3.9	18
Coffee creamer, liquid (1 Tbsp.)	20	68	1.5	1.4	0
Coffee creamer, powder (1 tsp.)	11	57	0.7	.6	0
Croissant (1)	235	46	12.0	3.5	13
Cream pie (⅙ 9″ pie)	455	46	23.2	15.0	8
Egg nog (1 cup)	342	50	19.0	11.3	149
Fruit pies (⅙ 9″ pie)	405	40	18.0	4.6	0
Lemon meringue (⅙ 9″ pie)	355	36	14.2	4.3	143
Pound cake (1/17 loaf)	110	41	5.0	3.0	64
Ice cream, vanilla (1 cup)	269	48	14.3	8.9	59
Ice cream, vanilla rich (1 cup)	349	61	23.6	14.7	88
Ice cream, French vanilla (1 cup)	377	54	22.6	13.5	153
Whipped cream (1 Tbsp.)	10	75	0.1	.5	3
Cream of chicken soup (1 cup)	191	54	11.5	4.6	27
Cream of mushroom soup (1 cup)	205	60	13.7	5.1	20

OILS
(1 tablespoon—100 to 125 calories (11 to 14 grams of fat)

	Sat. fat (gm.)	Poly. fat (gm.)	Mono. fat (gm.)	Choles. (mg.)
Lard	5.0	1.4	5.8	12
Beef tallow	6.4	.5	5.3	14
Palm	6.7	1.3	5.0	0
Butter	7.1	.4	3.3	31
Cocoa butter	8.1	.4	4.5	0
Palm kernel	11.1	.2	1.5	0
Coconut	11.8	.2	.8	0

Other oils (olive, peanut, sunflower, safflower, soybean, corn, rapeseed) contain a similar amount of fat but are much lower in saturated fat and therefore are preferable (for limited use) to those listed above.

The Fat in Fast Food

You may be able to get in and out in a hurry, but that convenience tends to carry a price, as the following figures show. One deluxe burger and an order of french fries can serve up all the fat you should have in an entire day. We're not suggesting you avoid fast food entirely, but we do advise that it should not be considered a "break" you deserve every day. The following figures represent a sampling of various fast-food menus.

Food	Cal.	Total fat (gm.)	% Fat
Regular burger	255	9.8	36
Regular cheeseburger	307	14.1	41
Large burger	424	21.7	46
Large cheeseburger	524	30.7	53
Deluxe burger (sauce)	563	33.0	53
Fish sandwich	400	17.0	38
Fish sandwich with cheese	440	21.0	43
Oysters, breaded	460	19.0	37
Clams, breaded	465	25.0	48
Fish with batter	159	9.5	54
Regular hot dog	273	15.0	49
Large hot dog	518	30.0	52
Large hot dog with cheese	593	36.0	55
Large hot dog with chili	555	33.0	54
Fried chicken, drumstick	136	8.0	53
Fried chicken, thigh	276	19.0	62
Fried chicken, wing	151	10.0	60
Bean burrito	343	12.0	31
Beef burrito	466	21.0	41
Beef tostada	291	15.0	46
Super burrito	457	22.0	43
Taco	186	8.0	39
Beans and cheese	168	5.0	27
French fries	214	10.0	42
Hush puppies	158	7.0	40
Coleslaw	138	8.0	52
Pizza, thin crust, cheese	450	15.0	30
Pizza, thick crust, cheese	560	14.0	23

Getting Over the Flavor of Fat

If you're feeling a little depressed at this point that lipo-fitness may have
to be "lipo-funless," keep the chin up. You may have your favorite treats.
Follow the lipo-fitness game plan diligently and you may have them quite
often, in fact. That's the beauty of the lipo-fitness program. It's lean where
it really counts, so it leaves room for splurges. Better yet, even mini-
splurges will feel like maxi-splurges because your taste buds will be in
such great shape. Unspoiled by overdose, they will become very easily
pleased. They will learn to love what they once only liked. And they will
learn to go absolutely nuts over what they used to love. But more on that
in chapter 28, "Lipo-Fit and Lipo-Full."

25

The Pros and Cons of Protein

Stamford

Nihil nimus (Nothing in excess).
—Latin proverb

Protein. We think so highly of the stuff that we now want it in our hair products, skin creams, and even stain removers.

But guess what, America. Whatever protein may be able to do for the living room carpet, as a component in the average American diet it's been a double-edged sword, a gift in the tradition of the Trojan horse. We view protein as a health ally, but all too often it comes to us filled with the very enemy we need to avoid most—saturated fat.

Think about it. We declare fat as our number one villain, but what's been making fat so prevalent in our diets in the first place? What's been behind the saying that meat builds strength, that crackers need cheese, and that a breakfast without eggs just isn't a real breakfast?

It's been protein—wily but worshipped protein. Some protein is absolutely essential, but many Americans get triple the amount needed. Add the fact that most of this protein is coming in foods that are over 50 percent fat, and you can see where the protein mystique has hurt more than it's helped.

A survey by the National Cancer Institute in 1984 determined that the top five sources of fat in the American diet were:

1. Ground beef products, including hamburgers, cheeseburgers, and meatloaf
2. Processed meats, including hot dogs and luncheon meats
3. Whole milk and whole milk drinks such as milkshakes
4. Doughnuts, cookies, and cakes
5. Beef steaks and roasts

With the exception of the baked goods, what are we looking at here?

We're looking at our protein "staples"—staples, unfortunately, that are punching holes in our health. It's not easy for me to malign protein like this, because for years I worshipped the stuff, too. When I was trying to build muscle by lifting weights in my teens and early twenties, I would whip up a milkshake that included whole milk, high-protein powder, ice cream, six eggs, and peanut butter.

Was I trying to build up my biceps with this monstrosity or the insides of my arteries?

The concoctions contained fewer calories from protein than fat, but the same unhealthy arithmetic plagues the majority of our most common protein sources. A hot dog, for example, is over 80 percent fat, and ground beef can be as high as 70 percent fat. Most cheeses are over 70 percent fat, and eggs are 68 percent fat. Even good old whole milk—"fitness you can drink"—is 48 percent fat. (We're speaking percentages of calories here.) Worse yet, the majority of the fat in these foods is saturated fat, the kind we need to avoid most of all.

But the fat aside, too much protein can pose problems in its own right. Research shows that excessive protein can be a risk factor for osteoporosis—weakening of the bones—as by-products of protein digestion can bind with calcium, which then gets lost in the urine. These by-products of protein digestion also can put undue stress on the kidneys and liver, especially with the onset of age. Because large amounts of water are needed to accomplish the considerable waste removal associated with protein digestion, excess protein also can increase risks of dehydration, especially in people who exercise heavily. The dehydrating effect of excessive protein is why high-protein diets can give the appearance of producing such rapid weight loss. The only thing being lost in the first few days is water. Nor is there anything special about protein's calories, as excess calories from protein merely get turned to fat just like any other calories eaten in excess of energy requirements.

Are we calling for a protein embargo here?

Absolutely not. Protein is a critical component of a healthy diet, responsible for far more than just healthy muscles. Protein helps bolster the immune system, keeps the nervous system intact, aids wound healing, contributes to healthy skin and hair, and even aids the digestive process by helping the body break down and absorb vital nutrients.

All we're calling for is balance. Just as the "more is better" argument got out of hand with aerobic exercise in this country, our approach to protein has been guilty of the same faulty logic. The average person needs no more than about 50 to 65 grams of protein a day, an amount satisfied by two glasses of skim milk and a 6 1/2-ounce can of tuna. To go considerably beyond this amount merely increases the likelihood that too much dietary fat will be consumed. Calcium loss and liver and kidney strain also can occur with excessive protein intake.

Stamford Answers "the Beef"

If all of this is striking you as a little hard to swallow, you might be wondering how Mother Nature could have allowed such a major flaw to occur in the first place. If protein is essential and saturated fat is nothing but harmful, why would she have made the two such frequent partners?

She didn't. We did. Virtually all of our protein foods highest in saturated fat are of our own making, processed meats such as those hot dogs, for example, and cheese. It could even be argued that whole milk was not part of Mother Nature's original plan, as the milking cow has been around for only about 3,000 years—a drop in the bucket compared to the 250,000-year history of our species as we currently know it.

But what about meat as it comes straight from the animal? There certainly couldn't be anything man-made or unnatural about a steak or a pork chop, right?

Wrong. There are lots of meat-eaters in the Louisville area, and I frequently get questions from readers of my weekly newspaper column, "The Body Shop," on just this subject. They want to know how meat can be a less than ideal source of protein if in fact it was, as most anthropologists acknowledge, the principal source of protein throughout our prehistoric past.

My answer: The animals eaten for their meat back then were as low in fat as the people stalking them. Warthogs, caribou, elk, bison, and even those wooly mammoths were lean and mean compared to the overfed and underexercised cattle and pigs that we eat today. The diets and activity levels of most livestock today are manipulated specifically with fat as the goal, because fat means greater tenderness and hence juicier prices.

A prime cut of beef today, at about 60 percent fat, serves up over three times as much fat as a comparable cut of wild bison, and even the leanest cuts of beef today, at nearly 30 percent fat, contain much more fat than our meats of old. In fattening our livestock, we've fattened ourselves.

When I made this information known in my column, it wasn't long before I received a letter from spokesmen for the beef industry. I was all wrong, they told me. Top round steak was only 9 percent fat, if trimmed and served broiled.

To which, as politely as I could, I had to answer "bull." I made it quite clear that a 3-ounce portion of top round, good for 162 calories and 5 grams of fat, offered 28 percent of its calories as fat. The math involved in that determination is very simple, as you'll recall from our last chapter. You multiply the number of grams of fat (5) times the number of calories a gram of fat contains (9) and get 45. Dividing 45 by 162, to get percent of calories from fat, produces 28 percent.

Where had the beef people gotten their fat figure of 9 percent?

Top round is 9 percent fat *by weight*, but that's not the way the American Heart Association has asked us to play the fat-calculating game. The AHA's recommendation for limiting fat intake to less than 30 percent is based on *percent of calories from fat* and not fat by weight. The dairy industry, as we mentioned, attempts to pull the same punch with its claim that whole milk is less than 4 percent fat. That's by weight. In terms of percent of calories from fat, whole milk is 48 percent fat. If you're a milk lover, as well you should be because milk is a great source of calcium as well as protein, drink skim milk or "1 percent fat" milk. In terms of calories, they are 5 percent and 22 percent fat, respectively, and just as nutrient rich. When milk is skimmed, it's skimmed of its fat only.

The Lipo-Fitness Promise

But enough on the cons of proteins. The stuff abounds with pros. It's the raw material of life itself, so let's learn to get it in a manner befitting that excellence, which means without a lot of fat. And let's also learn not to diminish the nutritional worth of protein by getting too much. Why turn Dr. Jekyll into Mr. Hyde through overdose?

Low-fat protein foods, along with complex carbohydrates, which you'll be learning about in our next chapter, have what it takes to form the pillars of what we're going to call "the lipo-fitness promise." The promise states: *"Eat foods that, in addition to being highly nutritious, also raise the body's metabolic rate, and you will lose body fat without having to reduce calories."*

At the heart of this promise is the phenomenon known as the Thermic Effect of Food (TEF), which we've discussed briefly in previous sections in this book. TEF refers to the amount of biochemical activity that certain foods require for digestion. The higher the TEF, the more calories the body needs to expend in order to break the food down and utilize its nutrients. The TEF for dietary fats, whether saturated or unsaturated, is very low—only about 3 percent of calories ingested, which is why dietary fats are so fattening. Almost nothing gets contributed to help fuel the body's digestive machinery. Studies with rats have shown that those fed high-fat meals show such small increases in metabolic activity as measured by increases in body heat that the animals appear almost to be on a fast.

Not so with low-fat protein foods, however, and to a lesser degree carbohydrates. The body can't store protein as protein, and the storage capacity for carbohydrate is small. The result is a dieter's dream come true—a substantial increase in metabolic rate (calorie-burning) as the body runs these foods through its digestive mill.

The energy required to break down, digest, and absorb protein comes to approximately one-fourth of the calories protein contains. Eat four scallops, in other words, and you essentially get one free. The energy required to break down carbohydrates is not that high, but it's higher than fat, and it increases when the carbohydrate intake increases and the storage capacity for carbohyrates has been met.

The Thermic Effect of Food is very real and has been the basis of some very worthwhile weight-loss programs introduced in the past few years. To get an idea of the impact the TEF phenomenon can have over an extended period, consider that merely by switching from a 40 percent fat diet (the current national average) to a 20 percent fat diet (the level we recommend in this book), the average person can lose body fat *without cutting back on calories*. Simply boosting the metabolic rate a few percent for several hours each day could easily save 25 calories, or 9,125 a year. One pound of fat is 3,500 stored calories, and thus 2.6 pounds of fat could be lost in one year from this change alone. And if you developed the habit of taking a walk after meals, you could double this effect.

But the best news is . . . *no deprivation*. In terms of sheer bulk, a switch away from fat in the diet can allow considerably greater food consumption, because low-fat foods are much lighter in calorie content. As an example, to get the same amount of fat contained in an average fast-food superburger with sauce, you would have to eat *all* of the following: a half pound of broiled chicken, 4 ounces of a low-fat fish such as haddock, six scallops, an entire head of lettuce, an onion, a cup of kidney beans, a cup of brown rice, a pound of green beans, one sweet potato, an ear of corn, a cup of raisins, an orange, two red beets, four asparagus spears, a half pound of peas (in their pods), a cup of popcorn, a cup of cooked spaghetti, and two slices of whole-wheat bread. (These calculations came from *The Natural Healing Cookbook*, by Mark Bricklin and Sharon Claussens, Rodale Press, 1981.)

Now that's a sandwich!

Don't think that a fast-food superburger is such a rare abomination, however, as two hot dogs or a couple of Danish pastries have similarly high fat contents.

We could indeed eat like kings if we could learn to get our proteins with less fat. To help you do that, may we offer the following information. Consider the chart "Who's Who in Proteins." Foods in Category One are your best protein sources because they contain the least amount of fat of all; foods in Category Two should be considered acceptable in moderation; and foods in Category Three should be restricted to once in a blue moon.

Keep the majority of your protein foods in Category One and you'll be making a huge step toward a lipo-fit body as well as lipo-fit blood. And do not be put off by the fact that many of the protein foods we permit are above the lipo-fitness limit of 20 percent fat. Protein should be making up only about 15 to 20 percent of your total caloric intake, remember, so the other lower-fat and carbohydrate foods you will be eating will be more than enough to keep you within the 20 percent lipo-fit goal.

Who's Who in Proteins: Separating the Lean from the Mean*

CATEGORY ONE—The Good
(less than 30% of total calories from fat)

Food	Cal.	Fat (gm.)	Sat. fat (gm.)	Mono fat (gm.)	Poly fat (gm.)	% Cal. from fat
Cottage cheese (½ cup, low-fat—2% fat by weight, 16 gm. protein)	101	2	1.4	.6	.07	18
Beef (top round) (3 oz., *lean only*, broiled, 27 gm. protein)	162	5	1.8	2.1	.25	28
Milk (skim) (1 cup, 8 gm. protein; "1% milk"—fat by wt. is 22% fat)	86	.4	.3	.1	trace	5
Chicken (½ breast, broiler or fryer, no skin, roasted, 27 gm. protein)	142	3	.9	1.1	.7	19
Fish (Atlantic cod) (3 oz., 19 gm. protein)	89	.5	.1	.1	.3	5
Fish (haddock) (3 oz., 21 gm. protein)	95	.5	.1	.1	.3	5

Lean only—means all visible fat is removed prior to eating.
Lean and fat—means food was prepared and eaten with fat that could have been removed remaining on meat.

Food	Cal.	Fat (gm.)	Sat. fat (gm.)	Mono fat (gm.)	Poly fat (gm.)	% Cal. from fat
Fish (perch) (3 oz., 20 gm. protein)	103	1.5	.2	.7	.5	13
Fish (tuna) (3 oz., canned in water, 23 gm. protein)	116	2	.6	.6	.8	16
Turkey (3 oz., light meat—no skin, roasted, 31 gm. protein)	145	1.2	.4	.2	.3	8

CATEGORY TWO—The O.K.
(31–45% of total calories from fat)

Food	Cal.	Fat (gm.)	Sat. fat (gm.)	Mono. fat (gm.)	Poly. fat (gm.)	% Cal. from fat
Cottage cheese (½ cup, 4.5% fat by weight, 14 gm. protein)	117	5	3.2	1.5	.2	38
Beef (3 oz., chuck, arm pot roast, *lean only*, braised, 28 gm. protein)	196	9	3.2	3.7	.3	41
Beef (3 oz., short loin, T-bone steak, *lean only*, broiled, 24 gm. protein)	182	9	3.5	3.5	.3	44
Lean ham (pork) (3 oz., leg, rump, roasted, 25 gm. protein)	187	9	3.1	4.1	1.1	43
Cured ham (pork) (3 oz., cured, boneless, extra lean—5% fat by wt., 18 gm. protein)	123	5	1.5	2.2	.5	37
Milk (low-fat) (1 cup, 2% fat by wt., 8 gm. protein)	121	5	2.9	1.4	.2	37
Chicken (1 leg, broiler or fryer, meat only—no skin, roasted, 26 gm. protein)	182	8	2.2	2.9	1.9	40
Chicken (½ breast, broiler or fryer, meat and skin, roasted, 29 gm. protein)	193	8	2.2	2.9	1.6	37
Fish (salmon) (3 oz., canned, drained solids with bone, 18 gm. protein)	120	5	1.2	1.6	1.3	38
Fish (tuna) (3 oz., canned in oil, drained solids, 23 gm. protein)	158	7	NA	NA	NA	40
Turkey (3 oz., dark meat and skin, roasted, 29 gm. protein)	193	7.5	2.2	2.4	1.9	35

CATEGORY THREE—The Ugly
(51% or more of total calories from fat)

Food	Cal.	Fat (gm.)	Sat. fat (gm.)	Mono. fat (gm.)	Poly. fat (gm.)	% Cal. from fat
Beef (3 oz., chuck, arm pot roast, *lean and fat*, braised, 23 gm. protein)	297	22	9.1	9.9	.9	67

Food	Cal.	Fat (gm.)	Sat. fat (gm.)	Mono. fat (gm.)	Poly. fat (gm.)	% Cal. from fat
Beef	204	12	4.9	5.1	.4	53
(3 oz., rib, whole—6–12 ribs, *lean only*, roasted, 23 gm. protein)						
Beef	324	27	11.4	12.1	.9	75
(3 oz., rib, whole—6–12 ribs, *lean and fat*, roasted, 19 gm. protein)						
Beef	276	21	8.7	9.1	.8	68
(3 oz., short loin, T-bone steak, *lean only*, broiled, 20 gm. protein)						
Lean ground beef	231	16	6.2	6.9	.6	62
(3 oz., lean—18% fat by wt., broiled, 21 gm. protein)						
Reg. ground beef	246	18	6.9	7.7	.7	66
(3 oz., regular—21% fat by wt., broiled, 20 gm. protein)						
Beef, processed (bologna, salami, frankfurters)—see "Fat Villains" table in chapter 24.						
Ham (pork)	233	15	5.5	6.9	1.7	58
(3 oz., leg, rump, *lean and fat*, roasted, 23 gm. protein)						
Pork, processed (bratwurst, salami, sausage, bacon)—see "Fat Villains" table in chapter 24.						
Egg, chicken	79	6	1.7	2.2	.7	68
(1 whole, 6 gm. protein)						
Milk, whole	150	8	5.1	2.6	.3	48
(1 cup, 3.3% fat by wt., 8 gm. protein)						
Chicken, processed (frankfurters)—see "Fat Villains" table in chapter 24.						
Chicken	285	16	4.4	6.4	3.7	51
(entire leg, broiler or fryer, meat and skin, fried, flour-coated, 30 gm. protein)						
Chicken	430	27	7.0	10.9	6.3	57
(drumstick and thigh, dark meat and skin, breaded and fried, 30 gm. protein)						
Chicken	494	30	7.8	12.2	6.8	55
(breast and wing, light meat, breaded and fried, 36 gm. protein)						
Chicken	515	29	8.5	10.4	8.4	51
(chicken fillet sandwich, plain, from fast-food restaurant, 24 gm. protein)						
Cheeses, hard (solid at room temperature)—see "Fat Villains" table in chapter 24.						
Turkey, processed (frankfurters, bologna)—see "Fat Villains" table in chapter 24.						

26

An Apology to Carbohydrate

Stamford

*Here is bread, which strengthens man's heart,
and therefore called the staff of life.*
—Matthew Henry, 1662–1714

I was having lunch the other day with a friend of mine who's trying
to lose about 15 pounds.

"What'll it be, gentlemen?" the waitress asked.

I was still undecided because I don't eat out very often and I had
never eaten at this place, but my friend had his order on the top of his
tongue. "I'll have the flame-broiled hamburger, without a roll, please, and
a tossed salad with Russian dressing."

Realizing suddenly that a point needed to be made, I ordered a bowl
of vegetable soup, two baked potatoes, a salad with wine vinegar as a
dressing, and my friend's unwanted roll.

When the waitress left, looking puzzled, I gave my friend a quick
lesson in math, because he also appeared puzzled. I estimated that his
lunch (assuming the broiled burger was in the neighborhood of 6 ounces
and that he'd be getting about two tablespoons of dressing on his salad)
was worth about 650 calories, with well over 50 percent of these calories
from fat. But my lunch was only about 500 calories, with less than 20
percent of its calories from fat. My friend found these numbers hard to
believe, especially when the two meals arrived and his looked tiny compared
to mine.

"But look at all that starch," he said.

161

"Yeah, isn't it great," I answered.

Starches, also called complex carbohydrates, are among the healthiest foods we can eat, yet many people still view them as fattening, thanks to the totally fallacious claims made by the high-protein/high-fat diets that have come and gone by a variety of titles: *The Scarsdale Medical Diet, Calories Don't Count, Dr. Atkins' Diet, The Drinking Man's Diet.* Maybe you remember those diets. Maybe you wish you could forget them. The diets said eat all the protein and fat you want, but do not eat carbohydrates and you'll lose weight. *The Drinking Man's Diet* even allowed unlimited hard liquor. What these diets did not tell you, however, was that they would drain you of water, energy, and good spirits like a sponge. Porter tells me his mother's experience with *The Drinking Man's Diet* back in the sixties resulted in temporary weight loss but also a temporary drinking problem. It became *The Drinking Mom's Diet.*

To this day, Porter's mother continues to view carbohydrates as fattening. Like millions of Americans, she thinks of them as empty-calorie foods that "puff" up the body. Better to have eggs for breakfast than pancakes. Better to have pork chops for dinner than spaghetti. Better to have a piece of cheese than a piece of bread. To achieve lipo-fitness, you need to realize the utter absurdity of that way of thinking.

We'll be giving you a brief chemistry lesson in carbohydrates shortly, but first may I tell how a switch to more complex carbohydrates changed my own life?

When I was exercising strenuously for at least forty minutes, six days a week, I was in great shape, but you wouldn't have known it by my energy levels. If I wasn't actually working out, I was dragging. And I even dragged through a lot of my workouts, as I recall. Part of the reason, I now know, is that I was neglecting dietary starches. I was eating a lot of protein and a lot of fat, and I was even getting my share of foods high in refined sugar, but I was not getting the fuel that energizes the body best. Protein is available as a source of muscular energy, but the body would rather burn fats and carbohydrates. And fat, despite its abundant 9 calories per gram, takes a back seat to carbohydrates, which are better suited for muscular energy as well as mental energy. And complex carbohydrates (starches) are the best.

Had I been avoiding starches on purpose?

Subconsciously is probably the better word. Like Porter's mother, I had an image of starch foods as being white and puffy in a way that would make me puffy if I ate too many of them. I felt safer with meat for my strength and sugar for my energy. Little did I realize that starches were better suited for both these roles.

Starches are converted by muscles and the liver into glycogen, which is the body's favorite fuel for muscular activity, but starches also keep the body steadily supplied with glucose—blood sugar—which is the only fuel that can be used by the brain. This is why high-protein diets that are deficient in carbohydrates can cause such lethargy and mental confusion. Neither the brain nor the brawn are being given the fuel they need. Approximately 65 percent of my calories now come from complex carbohydrates—either from whole-grain cereals and breads, brown rice, potatoes, beans, whole-wheat pastas, or vegetables—and I have never felt stronger or more energetic or smarter in my entire life.

Carbohydrates Under the Microscope

First things first: Carbohydrates are not foods but rather molecules in foods. And they do not come in just one form, but rather at least sixteen. The cellulose that goes "crunch" in a piece of celery is a carbohydrate, but then so is the syrup you pour on your waffles. All carbohydrates consist of carbon, hydrogen, and oxygen, but as you can see, Mother Nature has arranged those atoms in some remarkably dissimilar ways.

To achieve lipo-fitness, we suggest getting about 65 percent of your calories from carbohydrates, but we're not talking about relying on bon bons and maple syrup. Depending on how you get your carbohydrates, in fact, you could wind up anywhere from lean and healthy to obese and undernourished. The secret is to get your carbohydrates from foods that also are rich in vital nutrients, and complex, as opposed to simple, carbohydrates tend to qualify for that job best.

Complex carbohydrates—because they are more complex in their molecular makeup—also tend to digest more slowly than simple carbohydrates, thus avoiding the insulin rush and what candy lovers call the "sugar blues." Maybe you've experienced the phenomenon yourself if you've ever eaten something sugary on an empty stomach. First a surge of energy, but then a headachy lull. Insulin is the reason. One of insulin's jobs is to keep the amount of sugar in the blood (called glucose) from rising to unhealthful levels. Insulin does this by escorting blood sugar out of the blood and into the cells. But when a blood sugar "flood" occurs, such as with the consumption of a candy bar on an empty stomach, a case of overkill results. The pancreas panics and releases too much insulin, the result being a blood sugar "washout" as the excess insulin clears sugar from the blood almost entirely. Complex carbohydrates tend to avoid this over-reaction by the pancreas because their greater molecular complexity helps them digest more slowly.

Most complex carbohydrates, that is. Complex carbohydrates that have had their fiber removed through refinement, such as white flour, can be digested almost as quickly as simple carbohydrates and hence also can trigger a large insulin response. It's best to get your complex carbohydrates in forms that are as close to natural as possible—real potatoes, not instant; brown rice, not white; whole-grain breads, not those made from flour that has been robbed of its nutrients and fiber in the mill.

And the same goes for simple carbohydrates, because they, too, come in refined as well as natural forms. Table sugar (sucrose), for example, is a highly refined version of sugar cane or sugar beets, just as corn syrup is a highly refined version of the sugar that occurs naturally in corn. Because table sugar and corn syrup have been so completely removed from their original sources, however, they bring nothing to the body but empty calories. The healthiest and most natural way to satisfy a sweet tooth is the way we did it for the thousands of years before the likes of the candy bar ever came to be—by eating fresh fruit. Not only does fruit offer vital nutrients, but the sugar in fruit, called fructose, is unique in that it does not require insulin to enter cells. Fructose also digests more slowly than other forms of sugar, and its digestion gets slowed even further by the pulp of the fruit that contains it. All things considered, fruit is an ideal snack food and can make an even finer dessert. Try a slice of watermelon instead of a bowl of ice cream sometime and see if you don't agree. The watermelon has less than one-sixth of the calories and none of the fat. It's also an excellent source of vitamin A, and it contains fiber.

More "Carbo" Wisdoms

Here are some more tips for getting maximum health benefits from adding more carbohydrates to your diet.

☐ *Pay attention to your bread choices.* For maximum nutrition and fiber, try to eat breads whose labels boast that they are "100% whole wheat" or "whole grain" or "stone ground." The ingredients should list whole-wheat or stone-ground whole-wheat flour. Beware of relying just on the term "whole wheat" in the name, however, because the words can simply mean that the breads are made "wholly" from wheat flour, even though most of the flour has been refined. If one of the first few ingredients listed is "enriched" wheat flour, you have white flour bread. Molasses often is what gives these breads their brownish color.

As for white bread, do not think that it's totally without virtue, but do realize that it's made from flour that has been bleached with an ammonia in addition to having most of its fiber and nutrients removed through milling. Some of these nutrients get reinstated through "enrichment," but not sufficiently to bring the flour back to its natural status.

As for the new "lite" breads boasting added fiber, they're superior to white bread in fiber content, but all things considered—taste included—they are not as worthwhile as breads that were never defibered in the first place. We'll be giving you some easy whole-grain bread and muffin recipes later.

☐ *Learn to love the potato for the potato.* Low in calories and virtually fat-free, potatoes abound with vitamin C, potassium, B vitamins, phosphorus, magnesium, and even some protein. Make french fries out of a medium-size, 110-calorie potato, however, and you've suddenly got 600 calories on your hands, 42 percent of them from fat. Potato chips are even worse, at over 60 percent fat. Baking and boiling are best, frying is worse. Mashing is acceptable, just so long as you go easy on the butter and/or milk. Potato salad made with mayonnaise gets very low marks, as do potatoes au gratin because of their cheese.

☐ *Pile up the pasta.* Pasta is another highly nutritious, low-fat complex carbohydrate, but as with the potato, do not ruin its virtues with high-fat sauces. Choose whole-wheat pastas for nutrition and fiber. Meatless tomato sauces are best. Creamy/cheesey sauces are worst.

☐ *Master the art of low-calorie snacking.* Because carbohydrate foods tend to be our favorite foods for snacking, we should say a word here about that all-American pastime. Snacking doesn't have to be unhealthful if you do it right. Most important to avoid are the "chips"—be they potato, corn, or cheese-flavored—that have been fried in oil and highly salted. Not only can you really not eat just one, but most are over 50 percent fat. Best for snacking are vegetable sticks—carrots, celery, fresh broccoli, green peppers, cauliflower, or even string beans. Popcorn, air-popped and flavored with something other than butter, also is a healthy choice. It has only about 23 calories for a whole cup, which means you could have five cups for the same number of calories that are in just ten potato chips. Popcorn also is a good source of fiber and contains very little fat (only about 13 percent) if popped dry and served without butter.

Pretzels?

Acceptable, especially if unsalted. "Hard" pretzels made without shortening are best because they contain almost no fat.

Cheese and crackers with maybe a little ring bologna?

Sorry, but this is supposed to be a snack, not a meal. If you need to eat like that, you should go to the kitchen and do it right. One of the biggest dietary mistakes we make in this country is to eat huge amounts of calories without paying adequate attention. It's a form of sensory overload that can lead to abdominal overload. Try to concentrate on what you eat, whether you're eating a pretzel or a piece of prime rib. Paying attention allows for maximum pleasure with minimum intake.

Best Complex Carbohydrate Foods (Starches)

The following foods should comprise the bulk of a lipo-fitness diet. They are low in calories and fat and rich in nutrients and fiber. Try to include at least one of these foods at every meal—more if possible. Your fiber goal should be to consume at least 20 to 30 grams a day of total fiber, some soluble and some insoluble (details in the next chapter). Insoluble fiber is easy to find, but you'll have to be on the lookout for soluble fiber. Foods with an (*) in the fiber column are an excellent source of soluble fiber. Foods from the vegetable and simple carbohydrates list that follows also may be included in meeting this fiber quota.

Food	Serving size	Cal.	Prot. (gm.)	Total carbo. (gm.)	Dietary fiber (gm.)
BREAKFAST CEREALS: Ready-to-eat					

All have fewer than 10 grams of sugar—natural or added—and fewer than 3 grams of total fat per ounce.

Food	Serving size	Cal.	Prot. (gm.)	Total carbo. (gm.)	Dietary fiber (gm.)
All-bran	1 oz. ⅓ cup	71	4	21	8.5*
Cheerios	1 oz. 1¼ cups	111	4	20	2.1
Corn Flakes	1 oz. 1¼ cups	110	2	24	0.5
40% Bran Flakes	1 oz. ¾ cup	93	4	22	4.5
Grape Nuts	1 oz. ¼ cup	101	3	23	2.2
Life	1 oz. ⅔ cup	104	5	20	1.2
Raisin Bran	1.3 oz. ¾ cup	115	4	28	3.6
Shredded Wheat	1 oz. ¾ cup	115	4	25	3.9
Wheaties	1 oz. 1 cup	99	3	23	2.6

---

*Excellent source of soluble fiber; contains approximately 1 to 2 grams per serving.

Food	Serving size	Cal.	Prot. (gm.)	Total carbo. (gm.)	Dietary fiber (gm.)
CEREALS: Cooked					
(None have added sugar; all have fewer than 3 grams of fat per serving size stated.)					
Cream of Wheat, regular	1 cup	134	4	28	1.1
Oatmeal	1 cup	145	6	25	3.5*
Whole Wheat	1 cup	151	5	33	0.09
LEGUMES AND LEGUME PRODUCTS					
(Fewer than 3 grams of total fat in serving size stated.)					
Beans, kidney, all types, cooked, boiled	½ cup	112	8	20	5.8*
Lima beans, baby, cooked, boiled	½ cup	115	7	21	4.4*
Pinto beans, cooked, boiled	½ cup	117	7	22	5.3*
Peas, split, cooked, boiled	½ cup	116	8	21	5.1*

Food	Serving size	Cal.	Prot. (gm.)	Total carbo. (gm.)	Dietary fiber (gm.)
BREAD					
(All have fewer than 3 grams of fat per serving.)					
American rye bread	1 slice	61	2	13	0.9
Raisin bread	1 slice	66	2	13	N/A
Pumpernickel	1 slice	79	3	17	4.3
White	1 slice	76	2	14	0.5
Whole-wheat	1 slice	61	3	12	1.4
GRAINS AND GRAIN PRODUCTS					
(All have 3 grams of fat or less per serving stated.)					
Barley, pearled, uncooked	⅓ cup (1 cup cooked)	233	5	52	8.0*
Bulgur, cooked	1 cup	227	8	47	N/A
Rice, long-grain brown, cooked, hot	1 cup	232	5	50	4.8

Food	Serving size	Cal.	Prot. (gm.)	Total carbo. (gm.)	Dietary fiber (gm.)
Rice, white, cooked, long-grain, hot	1 cup	223	4	50	0.2
Macaroni, enriched, cooked, firm, hot	1 cup	192	7	39	1.2
Macaroni, enriched, cooked, tender, hot	1 cup	155	5	32	N/A
Macaroni, cooked, enriched, tender, cold	1 cup	117	4	24	N/A
VEGETABLES					
Corn, yellow, boiled	½ cup	89	3	21	3.9*
Potato, white, baked, flesh and skin (4¾" long, 2⅓" diameter)	1	220	5	51	4.8*
Potato, white, baked flesh only (same size as above)	1	145	3	34	N/A
Potato, boiled, cooked without skin, flesh only (2½" diameter)	1	116	2	27	2.7*
Potato, sweet, baked in skin (5" long, 2" diameter)	1	118	2	28	2.6*

Best Lipo-Fit Vegetables

Feel free to eat any of the following any time, any place, and in virtually any amount. These vegetables are such valuable sources of vitamins and fiber—and so low in both calories and fat—that we can feel safe in giving you that kind of green light. Do not abuse this freedom, however, by burying these vegetables in butter, gravy, or other high fat sources.

Food	Serving size	Cal.	Carbo. (gm.)	Dietary fiber (gm.)	Vit. A (IU)	Vit. C (mg.)
Asparagus, cooked, boiled, drained	½ cup	22	4	2.07	750	18
Beans, mung, mature seeds, sprouted, raw	½ cup	16	3	1.6	10	7
Beans, snap, fresh, cooked, boiled, drained	½ cup	22	5	2.1	410	6
Broccoli, cooked, boiled, drained, chopped	½ cup	23	4	2.0	1100	49
Broccoli, raw, chopped	½ cup	12	2	2.5*	680	41
Brussels sprouts, cooked, boiled, drained	½ cup	30	7	3.9*	560	48
Cabbage, cooked, boiled, shredded, drained	½ cup	16	4	1.9	60	18
Cabbage, raw, shredded	½ cup	8	2	0.7	40	16
Carrots, cooked, boiled, drained, sliced	½ cup	35	8	2.3*	19150	1.8
Carrots, raw, shredded (¾ of one raw carrot)	½ cup	24	6	1.3	15470	5.1
Cauliflower, cooked, boiled, drained, 1" pieces	½ cup	15	3	1.6	90	34
Cauliflower, raw	3 flowerets	13	3	1.8*	90	40
Celery, raw	1 stalk	9	2	1.3	510	3
Collards, cooked, boiled, drained, chopped	½ cup	13	3	2.2	2110	9.3
Cucumbers, raw, slices	½ cup	7	2	0.5	20	2.4
Eggplants, cooked, boiled, drained, 1" cubes	½ cup	13	3	2.0	30	0.6
Kale, frozen, cooked, boiled, drained, chopped	½ cup	20	3	2.3	4130	16.4

Food	Serving size	Cal.	Carbo. (gm.)	Dietary fiber (gm.)	Vit. A (IU)	Vit. C (mg.)
Lettuce, loose leaf, shredded	½ cup	5	1	0.6	530	5
Mushrooms, raw, pieces	½ cup	9	2	0.9	0	1.2
Okra, cooked, sliced	½ cup	25	6	2.6	460	13
Onion, cooked, boiled, drained, chopped	½ cup	29	7	2.2	0	6
Parsley, raw	10 sprigs	3	<1	0.4	520	9
Peas, green, frozen, cooked, boiled, drained	½ cup	63	11	4.6*	530	8
Peas, green, raw	½ cup	63	11	4.2*	500	31
Pepper, green, raw, chopped	½ cup	12	3	0.8	260	64
Spinach, cooked, boiled, drained	½ cup	21	3	2.0	7370	9
Spinach, raw, chopped	½ cup	6	1	0.7	1880	8
Squash, summer, cooked, slices	½ cup	18	4	0.7	260	5
Squash, summer, raw, slices	½ cup	13	3	0.7	130	10
Squash, winter, cooked, cubes	½ cup	57	15	3.6	440	11
Tomato, red, ripe, cooked, boiled	½ cup	30	7	1.0	1620	25
Tomato, raw (2⅗″ inches in diameter)	1 medium	24	5	0.8	1390	32
Turnip greens, cooked, boiled, drained	½ cup	15	3	2.8	3960	20

Best Simple Carbohydrate Foods (Sugars)

Not all sugars are evil. The following fruits, despite containing the simple sugar fructose, supply fiber and vital nutrients, and they also are virtually devoid of fat. No "hollow" calories here. They can satisfy a sweet tooth with style, so eat them with meals, as desserts, or as a snack.

Food	Serving size	Cal.	Carbo. (gm.)	Dietary fiber (gm.)	Vit. A (IU)	Vit. C (mg.)
Apple, raw, without skin (2¾" diameter)	1	72	19	2.6	60	5
Apple, raw, with skin (2¾" diameter)	1	81	21	2.8	70	8
Apple juice, canned or bottled	1 cup	116	29	1.5	0	2
Banana, raw (8¾" long, 1¹³⁄₃₂" diameter)	1	105	27	2.0	90	10
Blackberries, raw	½ cup	37	9	4.5	120	15
Blueberries, raw	½ cup	41	10	2.5	70	9
Dates, dried	10 dates	228	61	8.0	40	0
Figs, dried, uncooked	1 fig	48	12	3.7	30	0
Grapefruit, raw	½	38	10	1.7	150	41
Grapes, raw, American type (slip skin)	10	15	4	0.5	20	1
Grapes, raw, European type (adherent skin)	10	36	9	0.5	40	5
Melon, cantaloupe, raw	¼ small	57	13	1.6	5160	68
Melon, honeydew, raw, cubed	1 cup	60	16	1.5	70	42
Orange juice, raw	1 cup	111	26	0.75	500	124
Orange, raw (2⅝" diameter)	1	62	15	1.95	270	70
Peach, raw (2½" diameter)	1	37	10	1.39	910	11
Pear, raw Bartlett (2½" diameter, 3½" long)	1	98	25	5.0	30	6.6
Pineapple, raw, diced pieces	½ cup	39	10	1.2	20	12
Plums, raw (2⅛")	1	36	9	1.4	210	6
Prunes, dried, uncooked	10	201	53	13.5	1670	2.8

Food	Serving size	Cal.	Carbo. (gm.)	Dietary fiber (gm.)	Vit. A (IU)	Vit. C (mg.)
Raisins, seedless, packed	¼ cup	123	33	2.7	30	1
Strawberries, raw	1 cup	45	10	3.3	40	85
Watermelon, diced	1 cup	50	11	1.4	580	15

Foods for a Fit Electrical System

The human body may consist of flesh and blood, and carbohydrates may be its favorite fuel, but electricity runs the show. Electrical impulses trigger the beating of the heart, the flexing of the skeletal muscles, the functioning of the nervous system and brain, even the process called "mineralization," which keeps bones strong. Virtually every cellular interaction that goes on in the body—and there are billions every second—depends on a flow of electricity.

What generates this electricity?

The interaction of chemicals. Just as the interaction of chemicals can create an electrical charge in a battery, chemical interactions create electrical impulses in the body, and crucial for the proper transmission of these electrical impulses are certain dietary minerals known as "electrolytes." Maybe you've heard the term in connection with certain athletic beverages. This is because heavy sweating can deplete the body of electrolytes, which these beverages are designed to help replace.

But electrolytes are important for all of us, not just hard-exercising athletes, and two electrolytes—potassium and calcium—appear to be especially vital for their ability to reduce blood pressure and hence reduce risks of both heart attacks and strokes. The exact mechanisms by which these minerals exert their influence remain uncertain, but researchers speculate that they help the body deal with excess sodium and that they also may be involved directly with the electrical impulses responsible for blood vessel constriction (and hence hypertension) in the first place. In one research study, a single daily serving of a potassium-rich fruit or vegetable was found to reduce risks of stroke over a twelve-year period by 40 percent. The protection occurred, moreover, whether blood pressure came down or not.

Calcium's antihypertensive talents have been demonstrated in studies involving people with high blood pressure who have been found to be calcium-deficient. Bringing calcium levels up invariably brings blood pressure down. Considering calcium's abilities to protect against osteoporosis (weakening of the bones) and cancer of the colon as well, it's a nutrient not to be slighted.

But slighted it has been, as has potassium. Surveys show that as many as half of U.S. adults may not get the Recommended Daily Allowance (RDA) for calcium (1,000 mg.) and that our reduced consumption of fresh fruit (down 43 percent since 1930) may have our potassium intakes below healthful levels also. Some nutritionists feel we should be getting as much as 8,000 to 10,000 mg. of potassium daily, but a diet short on fruits and vegetables would be hard-pressd to produce one-fifth that much.

Will you be covered for these two vital nutrients on our lipo-fitness program?

Absolutely. Fruits and vegetables are your best potassium sources and low-fat dairy products, fish, and some vegetables are excellent sources of calcium. We include the following information to assist you in making sure your intakes of these important minerals are adequate. Remember: You should be getting at least 1,000 mg. a day of calcium and between 5,000 and 10,000 mg. daily of potassium.

Best Low-Fat Sources of Calcium

Food (portion size)	Calcium (mg.)
Broccoli, cooked (½ cup)	89
Blackstrap molasses (1 Tbsp.)	137
Brussels sprouts, cooked (1 cup)	56
Chickpeas, dried (¼ cup)	75
Collards, cooked (½ cup)	74
Cottage cheese, low-fat (½ cup)	80
Dandelion greens, cooked (½ cup)	73
English muffin (1)	96
Figs, dried (10)	269
Great Northern beans, cooked (1 cup)	90
Ice milk (1 cup)	176
Kale, cooked (½ cup)	47
Kidney beans, canned (1 cup)	74
Milk, skim (1 cup)	302
Mustard greens, cooked (½ cup)	52
Navy beans, cooked (½ cup)	48
Okra, cooked (½ cup)	88
Orange (1 whole)	52
Oysters (1 cup)	120
Pinto beans, cooked (1 cup)	86
Prunes, dried, pitted (10)	43

Food (portion size)	Calcium (mg.)
Raisins (1 cup)	71
Rhubarb (1 cup)	348
Salmon, sockeye (3 oz.)	210
Sardines, Atlantic (3 oz.)	372
Scallops, steamed (3 oz.)	109
Shrimp (3½ oz.)	320
Spinach, cooked (1 cup)	244
Soybeans (½ cup)	131
Turnip greens, cooked (1 cup)	198
Yogurt, low-fat (1 cup)	448

Hard cheese is an excellent source of calcium, containing between 400 and 500 mg. per ounce for most varieties, but high fat content (about 70 percent of calories) makes hard cheeses a less desirable calcium food than these other lower-fat sources. Whole milk also is an excellent calcium source, but so is skim and low-fat milk, with a lot less fat.

Best Low-Fat Sources of Potassium

Food (portion size)	Potassium (mg.)
Apple (1 whole)	159
Apricots, fresh (3)	313
Banana (1 medium)	451
Blackberries, raw (1 cup)	282
Blackstrap molasses (1 Tbsp.)	585
Broccoli, cooked (½ cup)	127
Cantaloupe, (¼)	413
Cherries, raw (10)	152
Chicken, light meat (3 oz.)	187
Cod (3 oz.)	323
Cottage cheese, low-fat (1 cup)	217
Dates, whole (10)	541
Figs, dried (10)	1331
Flounder (3 oz.)	498
Grapefruit, raw (½)	158
Grape Juice, bottled (1 cup)	334
Great Northern beans (½ cup)	374

Food (portion size)	Potassium (mg.)
Haddock (3 oz.)	297
Ice milk (1 cup)	265
Milk, skim (1 cup)	406
Navy beans, cooked (½ cup)	395
Nectarine, raw (1)	288
Orange, raw (1 whole)	237
Orange juice (1 cup)	496
Pear, raw (1 whole)	208
Perch, (3 oz.)	243
Pineapple, raw chunks (1 cup)	175
Potato, baked (1 large)	844
Prunes, dried uncooked (10)	626
Raisins (½ cup)	545
Rhubarb, cooked (1 cup)	230
Round steak, trimmed of fat (3 oz.)	297
Salmon (3 oz.)	378
Sardines, Atlantic (3 oz.)	501
Scallops, steamed (3 oz.)	405
Soybeans, cooked (½ cup)	486
Squash, winter, cooked (½ cup)	445
Strawberries, raw (1 cup)	247
Sweet potato, baked (1)	397
Tomato (1)	254
Tuna, drained (3 oz.)	225
Turkey, light meat (3 oz.)	259
Yogurt, low-fat (1 cup)	573

27

Fabulous Fiber: Different Types for Different Gripes

Stamford

Oats. A grain, which in England is generally given to horses, but in Scotland supports the people.
— Samuel Johnson, 1709–1784

Just what is this stuff called fiber, and where does it fit into the lipofitness game plan?

Fiber is a type of nondigestible complex carbohydrate, and it needs to be a much busier player than it has been. The average American today, despite all the recent fiber fanfare, consumes only about a third of the 20 to 30 grams of daily fiber our digestive systems may optimally require. This has been due partly to our reduced consumption of fruits and vegetables, which are rich fiber sources, but food processing also must shoulder the blame. The milling of most whole grains—wheat included—reduces their fiber content by at least 50 percent. This allows the flours to bake into lighter and fluffier goods, but light and fluffy isn't what the human digestive system evolved on. For 250,000 years we ate roots, stems, and leaves, but now some of us resist even the crust on our white bread. Even as recently as 100 years ago we were getting far more fiber than we do today.

The result of this softening of the American diet?

Our intestines have been allowed to get out of shape. We think of technological progress as having its greatest impact on the deconditioning of our muscles and hearts, but it's clear that our bowels have been suffering from having things too easy as well. A diet deficient in indigestible roughage is a risk not just for constipation, but for hemorrhoids, diverticulosis, appendicitis, and colon cancer. "Use it or lose it" is a concept that applies to virtually every part of the human body. Here's a quick rundown of the disorders that may be avoided by getting sufficient intestinal exercise via a diet that contains adequate bulk.

☐ *Hemorrhoids*. Roughage (also called "insoluble" fiber because it does not dissolve in water, but rather absorbs water like a sponge) is found in the skins of fruits and vegetables, in grain products such as wheat bran, and in whole-grain cereals and bread. By giving bulk to the stools and also softening them, it acts as a laxative, thus reducing the likelihood of hemorrhoids (swollen rectal veins), which often result from excretional straining. There's evidence that dietary roughage may even help prevent varicose veins, which also can be aggravated by excessive bathroom toil.

☐ *Diverticulosis*. The same laxative effect that helps prevent hemorrhoids also can help prevent the bulging of the bowel into pockets, called diverticula, which can become inflamed and infected to the point of requiring surgery. A diet that keeps stools soft and free-moving prevents both the pressure that can create these bulges and the compacted waste that can infect them.

☐ *Appendicitis and colon cancer*. The cleansing action that roughage has on the intestinal tract also can reduce chances of bacterial infection that can be a risk for appendicitis, and it can reduce risks of colon cancer as well. Research suggests that cancerous activity in the large intestine may be instigated by mutagenic compounds in waste material that is allowed to remain in prolonged contact with bowel walls. A diet rich in insoluble fiber reduces this exposure time by keeping things moving.

☐ *Obesity*. Because insoluble fiber is by definition indigestible, it offers no calories, but it does offer feelings of fullness, so it's an ideal aid for weight loss. Insoluble fiber also can reduce the absorption of other calories, and fat calories especially, by accelerating food's movement through the gut. Some research indicates that a fiber-rich diet may reduce caloric absorption overall by as much as 3 percent, enough to account for 60 "free" calories a day on a 2,000-calorie-a-day regimen. Too much fiber, however, also may decrease the absorption of important vitamins and minerals, so the use of high-fiber supplements is not advised. Even wheat bran and oat bran should be used in moderation. You're best off getting your fiber in the amounts that occur in foods naturally.

Soluble Fiber

But there's more to the fiber story than just the indigestible roughage
that promotes fit intestines. There's another type that encourages fit blood
by lowering serum cholesterol. It's called soluble fiber, because it does
dissolve in water, and it's the component that's been behind the incredible
oat bran craze of the past few years. Despite all the hoopla, however, the
stuff does work. I'm convinced it's been instrumental in my own cholesterol
drop of over 100 points. I eat a big bowl of old-fashioned uncooked oatmeal
(no advantage over cooked—it's just quick and easy) every morning with
bananas or raisins or seasonal fruits such as peaches, blackberries, or
strawberries. I also eat a lot of beans, brown rice, fruits, and vegetables,
all of which are also good sources of soluble fiber.

But how can something that works in the intestines wind up affecting
cholesterol in the blood?

The answer lies in a yellowish green liquid secreted by the liver, bile.
Bile's purpose is to help with the digestion of fats, and it's pretty precious
stuff. It's precious enough for the body to use it over and over, in fact.
Only a small amount gets lost each time it goes to work, the remainder
getting reabsorbed through the intestinal walls and stored in the gall
bladder.

Unless one eats a lot of soluble fiber, that is. Soluble fiber mixes with
water to form a gel (look for it the next time you eat cooked oatmeal)
that coats the intestinal walls and prevents bile from being reabsorbed.
This forces the body to make new bile.

And what's the principal raw material from which bile is made?

Cholesterol. The need for new bile persuades the body to pull cholesterol out of the blood, and hence levels tend to come down. Some
cholesterol-lowering drugs work in this same way, but certainly not as
safely, nutritiously, or as cheaply as oats. (A recent research study reported
that the amount of oat bran needed to lower cholesterol significantly in
one year would cost less than 18 percent of a year's supply of the leading
cholesterol-lowering medication.)

Before you get too excited about oat bran, however, realize that there
are good and bad ways to get it. One gentleman who came to me for advice
in lowering his cholesterol made the mistake of eating huge portions of
a certain crunchy and very tasty oat bran cereal each day, only to see his
cholesterol rise by 30 points in six months. The cereal, as it turned out,
had only a trace of oats and very little soluble fiber. What it did have,
however, was plenty of coconut oil, and hence saturated fat, the worst
kind for raising cholesterol. Keep this man's experience in mind when
shopping. Just because a product contains oat bran doesn't mean it contains enough to do any good, especially if the other ingredients in the
product supply dietary fat.

Nor should you think that oats are the only good source of cholesterol-lowering soluble fiber. Research recently has found rice bran to be a rich source of soluble fiber. It's only in unprocessed brown rice, however, so don't go running to the market for something that's going to be ready in a minute. I strongly suspect that rice, as much as my morning bowl of oatmeal and other dietary changes, has helped in the reduction of my cholesterol. In addition to having brown rice with beans once or twice a week, I frequently have a dessert of brown rice pudding (made with skim milk). It's delicious, but be careful. It's pretty high in calories, and if you need to lose weight, you're better off to pass on this one. See our recipe section if you're interested.

Choose smart cereals. Smartest of all is good, old-fashioned oatmeal made from oats that have been "rolled" or "steel cut." Unlike instant oatmeal, which has lost some of its bran to less respectful forms of milling, rolled and steel-cut oats are left with more of their fibrous hulls intact. As for cold cereals, there are dozens of worthwhile options, so let your taste buds be your guide. Do try to avoid those with lots of added sugar, however, and do try to befriend a brand that's got some fiber. As for added vitamins and minerals, don't be overly impressed with brands that promise 100 percent of everything. Most cereals are fortified with at least 25 percent of what these super-cereals offer, and for considerably less money. (Porter tells me a favorite breakfast of his is wheat bran flakes sprinkled with oat bran, a combination that supplies soluble as well as insoluble fiber all in one bowl.)

A word on gas: Adding high-fiber foods to the diet may cause some intestinal discomfort and/or gas in the early going, but be patient. You may simply require a period of adaptation, as your intestinal chemistry needs time to get used to the change. If you find yourself overwhelmed, however, cut back and build your fiber intake back up gradually. Your goal, remember, should be to become comfortable with between 20 and 30 grams of fiber a day—some soluble, some insoluble. If this sounds excessive, keep in mind that some rural Africans get over 100 grams a day. My own intake is 50 grams or more a day, and I still have a social life.

Summary

The nutrition story is an intriguing one because it demonstrates once again how the fitness movement has tended to miss the point. Yes, a certain level of physical activity is important for good health, and yes, modern technology for many of us has taken that level of activity away.

But what else has modern technology taken away that has had perhaps an even greater impact on our health?

It's taken away our naturally healthful diets. It's taken the fiber out of our carbohydrates and it's put fat into our proteins. And it's put sugar and salt everywhere but where it belongs, which is in the kitchen sink. Jogging to Peru and back again isn't going to change any of that. The "sweat" that most of us need to invest is in returning to the kinds of foods that can build fitness on a cellular level, if not an athletic one. We need to get into shape from the inside out.

28

Lipo-Fit and Lipo-Full

Stamford

I can't believe I ate the whole thing.
—Alka-Seltzer commercial

Cave couple Bob and Helen haven't had a thing to eat in three days and it's beginning to make them cranky. Helen calls Bob a loser; he heaves his spear at a tree out of frustration, misses, but scores a bull's-eye on a warthog napping in a bush nearby.

Are Bob and Helen going to exercise dietary restraint, chew at least sixteen times before swallowing, and make sure to put their forks (hands) down between bites?

You and I might not be here right now if they had. Our rocky evolutionary road taught us to eat what we could when we could. Portion control meant making the portion as large as possible and eating it before someone else did. No wonder most weight-loss strategies have met with such dismal failure over the years. They violate our 250,000-year history of loving to eat.

"The classical and memorable meals of our prehistoric past were the two- and three-day massive 'pig-outs' following the successful capture of a wild boar, antelope, or zebra," write Bernhoff A. Dahl, M.D., and David Fingard, M.D., in their tongue-in-cheek and yet thought-provoking weight-loss book of the late seventies, *The Pig Out Diet*. "Vast fortunes have been made writing and preaching about diet schemes and social clubs for weight control, as well as by selling gadgets, postal scales for weighing out minuscule portions, drugs, and memberships. None of these approaches, however, deals with man's most basic nature—the urge to consume food abundantly whenever available."

Our problem now, of course, is that food is not just available, it's inescapable. It's as though our food now stalks us, thanks to the incessant advertising campaigns of everything from fast-food hamburgers to pizza guaranteed to be at your doorstep within thirty minutes. Making matters worse is the nature of this food. Were cave people Bob and Helen to sit down to a fast-food meal today, it's likely they'd have turned green with something other than envy.

The solution to our peril of plenty?

We've got to start thinking more about the quality of what we eat so that we can stop thinking about the quantity. We need, in other words, to be able to return to our "free-style" ways of old. We need to stop thinking that a full stomach has to become a fat stomach. We need to realize that foods low in fat and refined sugar may be eaten with the prehistoric abandon that still simmers in our genes. By centering your diet around the foods listed on the lipo-fitness menu, you may forget you ever knew what a calorie was. You may rediscover the joy of feeling full without feeling guilty. You may reintroduce the word "seconds" to your vocabulary.

The Healthy Splurge

Great, but where will the pleasure be? Who needs seconds on kidney beans and brown rice?

Lipo-fit foods allow considerably more fun and variety than that. What's more, you eat healthfully enough on the lipo-fitness menu that splurges become legal. And the splurges taste all that much better because you have gotten your taste buds in such great shape. One of the problems with the way many of us eat today is that we've spoiled our taste buds to the point of needing dietary disaster to get their attention.

People are shocked when they see me, Mr. Lipo-Fitness himself, "pig out" at restaurants and parties. What they fail to realize, however, is that I don't do it often—once every few weeks at most—and that I earn these sprees with the exceptionally healthy diet that I eat most of the time. The following numbers should help prove the "pudding" of which I speak:

- The average American adult eats between 80 and 90 grams of fat a day—roughly 800 calories worth, which comes to 5,600 for a week.
- The average American adult also eats about 20 teaspoons of refined sugar a day—about 360 calories worth, which comes to 2,520 for a week.

Add the two and you get 8,120 calories. That comes to 58 percent of the typical American's average weekly intake—quite a bit, considering that these calories are not just nutritionally empty but also directly harmful to the body in a variety of ways.

But what happens to this lofty figure when you eat lipo-fitly?

It gets cut by at least 60 percent—4,872 calories—which is great not just for health and weight control, but it's also great for people like me who like to splurge. By sitting down to a bowl of ice cream twice a week at roughly 500 calories per bowl, I still am cashing in on only 1,000 of those 4,872 "junk" calories that I've earned by eating lipo-fitly. Even by splurging every few weeks at a restaurant or party, I still am averaging far fewer empty calories a week than the 8,120 that most people consume routinely.

But won't such splurges raise Cain with the positive changes in serum cholesterol that a low-fat diet can achieve?

Research, as well as my own cholesterol, suggests not. If I splurge daily for a week or more I'll see a rise, but the occasional sprees seem to have little effect. Similar results were found in a study in which people on low-fat diets were fed "splurge" meals as often as once every other day. As long as the people otherwise kept to their low-fat regimens, the splurge meal (consisting of a ham and cheese sandwich and a milk shake) made no significant impact on their total cholesterol or LDL or HDL subfractions. This is consistent with our 80/20 policy. Assuming that six meals were consumed every two days, five good meals out of six means that 83 percent of the time the people in this study ate healthy low-fat food. Pigging out the other 17 percent of the time created no lasting negative effects.

The Healthy Gorge

But certainly the best news about taking the low-fat road is the sheer volume it allows you to eat. As Dr. Martin Katan boldly states in his 1989 best-seller *The T-Factor Diet,* "If you want to pig out occasionally with little danger of gaining fat weight, do it on carbohydrates."

Dr. Katan bases his statement on a study that found that the body is capable of handling occasional excesses of as many as 2,000 calories from carbohydrates without synthesizing or storing any of the calories as fat. The body bends over backwards to convert excess carbohydrate into glycogen, which it stores in the muscles and liver, before it will convert excess carbohydrate to fat. Two thousand calories, incidentally, is the amount in approximately fourteen bagels, or twenty baked potatoes, or twenty-eight ears of corn, or thirty-three slices of whole wheat bread, or thirty-five peaches, or sixty-six carrots, or eighty-seven cups of air-popped popcorn, or 588 grapes.

Get the idea?

If you like to eat, carbohydrates are the way.

Lipo-Fit Nibbling

And what if you're a nibbler?

That's fine on the lipo-fitness program, too, and even better for met-abolic reasons. Large meals, even if they're low in fat, tend to cause the release of more insulin than small meals, and insulin as you'll recall, tends to encourage calories to be stored as fat rather than burned for energy. Hence the weight-control advantages of eating lightly but often.

Notice the word "lightly," however. Snacking on such snack food staples as potato chips (60 percent fat) and nuts (80 to 90 percent fat) and cheese (70 percent fat) is not going to work. Try to keep your snacks as low in fat as the other foods on your lipo-fit menu. Good choices are air-popped popcorn, vegetable sticks, fresh fruit, or crackers such as matzoh or Swedish flat breads, made without vegetable oil or a lot of salt. Be careful with snacking, however, even if your snacks are healthful ones. There's a tendency to munch mindlessly, which can add up to more than you realize, and there's a tendency to undervalue the calories from snacks because they haven't come by way of an actual sit-down meal.

Our advice is to keep snacking to a minimum. Small meals are fine, but snacking between those meals may not be. Boredom rather than hunger is probably what's motivating you. If you're actually hungry, then prepare something that's going to impress you as being a meal. Then get out of the kitchen.

Getting Tough with the Taste Buds

"Sure, I love a baked potato, but don't ask me to eat it without butter or sour cream."

"Broccoli's great, as long as it's got enough hollandaise sauce."

"I could eat fish three nights a week—breaded and fried."

When I hear people talk like that, I don't know whether to get annoyed or feel sorry for them. Dietary fat is killing us of heart disease, cancer, diabetes, and strokes—in addition to making us fat—yet we can't lay off the stuff because we're at the beck and call of our taste buds. It doesn't say much for our priorities. Our waistlines are asking us to say no, our hearts are asking us to say no, our cancer-defense mechanisms are asking us to say no, and yet we say yes. "Why?" I ask these people.

"Because life's too short," is the usual response.

How much sense does that make? Life becomes too short *because* of the butter, sour cream, hollandaise sauce, and deep fryer. A high intake of fat—and saturated fat especially—is suspected of contributing to as many as two-thirds of all deaths from heart disease in the United States and as many as 45 percent of all deaths from cancer. Add its influences on the metabolic disorders responsible for diabetes, and its unfavorable effects on blood clotting that can lead to strokes, and you've got dietary fat as a major accomplice in four of our leading causes of death. Havoc like that can't be claimed by even the cigarette.

If I'm beginning to sound a little high and mighty here, I apologize, but remember that I, too, was once a slave to my taste buds. My enslavement was an extension of my dietary upbringing, for one thing, but it was made even worse by my belief that my excessive exercise habits were freeing me from any negative consequences. "Lean on the outside meant lean on the inside," I assumed, but I learned how wrong that was when I found my cholesterol was over 200. That's when it hit me that my whole orientation to health had been wrong, that exercise was not king, that it was little better than a court jester, in fact, fooling me into believing that I could have my healthy heart and ham and eggs, too. I was going to have to make a change and it scared me because food for me, as it may be for you, was a great pleasure as well as a great solace. I found it relieved stress, and was I now going to allow it to cause me stress?

Yes, I was. But unlike going "cold turkey," as I did in quitting my exercise addiction, I was going to take this one differently. I was going to go slowly. "Piece by peace" was going to be my motto. I started by avoiding fast-food lunches, and that was the only major change I made the first year. Then, influenced by my wife, Joy, I started reducing the fat in my diet at home.

How did I feel on my new low-fat plan?

Because I made changes gradually, I felt no deprivation at all. In the first year, I went from a diet that was probably 45 percent fat to one deriving only about 30 percent of its calories from fat. Since then I've dropped even lower—to about 20 percent fat—and without missing my old greasy favorites at all. Occasionally I'll have something high in fat just for old time's sake, and though I won't deny that it tastes heavenly, it leaves me feeling a little hellish. The reason, some digestive experts have explained to me, is that my fat-digesting mechanisms have in a sense gotten out of shape. A meal that used to be a piece of cake to digest now feels like a marathon. If I have something fatty for breakfast on Sunday morning at 10:00, I'll feel sluggish and even a little ill until late in the afternoon. I've talked to other people who've gotten away from fatty foods and they share my experience.

If Rats Can Do It, People Can

Sounds great, but you know your taste buds too well? There's no way a piece of broiled fish is going to satisfy you like a juicy sirloin?

Don't be so sure. Studies show that people can be made to forget all about their preferences for salt in just a few months. And if a recent experiment with rats is any indication, preferences for fat can be forgotten as well. Rats put on low-fat diets lost their appetites for fat in just two weeks. It's something to think about, certainly, as TV advertising insists upon convincing us there's simply no defense against the likes of a "Mac attack." The body adapts to find pleasure in whatever we give it. I can honestly say that I now look forward to sitting down to homemade bread and a bowl of bean soup as much as I ever did a plate of prime rib. Especially nice is that I can now look forward to indulging in such healthy gluttony with far greater frequency. Since what I now eat is much lower in fat and calories, it digests more quickly, thus readying me for my next meal in delightfully short order. I now eat four or five light meals a day, whereas I used to eat three heavies.

But the biggest reason to reduce dietary fat, of course, is health. Studies show that for every 1 percent that you can get your cholesterol to drop, your risks of heart disease drop by 2 percent. Add to that the inarguable weight-control advantages to avoiding fat, and the case against the stuff becomes air-tight. People in one study lost weight when allowed to eat all they wanted on a low-fat diet, but quickly began to gain weight as soon as fat content was raised to 45 percent of calories, which is only slightly higher than the current American average. This study, along with others, suggests that the human appetite is not good at judging appropriate caloric intake when fat content rises beyond a level of about 25 percent. The amount we need to eat to feel satisfied, purely from a standpoint of bulk, simply winds up representing too many calories on a high-fat regimen.

Worse yet, there is evidence that a history of high-fat eating can actually begin to change the way fat gets metabolized: A shift takes place toward fat being stored instead of being used for energy. The shift has to do with increased activity of an enzyme called lipoprotein lipase (LPL), whose job it is to break fat molecules down into components (called fatty acids) small enough to get through the walls of the body's fat cells. The more fat you eat, the more active this fat-storing enzyme becomes. Worse yet, the fatter you get, the more active this enzyme becomes. A doubly inflationary momentum can begin to build. Add a preference for sugar and you've really got trouble, because sugar also can substantially boost LPL activity. The combination   a high fat diet that's also high in refined sugar—is a fat-making duo tough to defeat. Sugar, by calling up insulin, gets the doors to fat cells swinging wide open, and a high-fat diet gives those open doors plenty to invite inside by loading the bloodstream with fat molecules. Add LPL as an all too accommodating desk clerk in this hotel analogy and the picture becomes complete. A diet high in both sugar and fat—which the typical American diet is—offers the fat-making process a luxury suite that it just can't pass up.

So maybe you're lamenting your sweet tooth now as much as your appreciation of a good white sauce? Rest assured that a sweet tooth, too, can be tamed. Witness the story of a primitive tribe living on an isolated tropical island whose initial reaction to an American candy bar was one of wrinkled noses. "Too sweet" was the verdict that got translated. And small wonder when you think about it. Nothing in the natural world has the concentration of refined sugar (sucrose) that resides in the likes of a Milky Way.

PART
IV

CLOSING REMARKS: PUSH-UPS FOR THE PERSONALITY

29

Health Takes Lessons from Happiness

Shimer

Strength through joy.
—Robert Ley, 1890–1945

When I was writing a newsletter called *Executive Fitness* for the business community back in the late seventies and early eighties, fully a third of the information I chose to report dealt with psychology rather than physical fitness. But no one ever complained. It must have been as clear to my readers as it was to me that the mind exerts considerable influence over physical health. When we're happy or unhappy, relaxed or stressed, content or worried, our bodies get the message and they respond in very specific ways. We need to keep this in mind as we chart out what may seem to be logical paths to good health. Any diet or exercise effort that puts undue stress on the mind is not going to be optimally healthy for the body. We need to value the comfort of whatever health steps we make as much as the physiological ground those steps may cover.

Baloney, you say. Health is a matter of biology pure and simple.

Maybe so, but the mind is responsible for how appropriately that biology behaves. Our bodies may fight the fight against disease, but how well they fight depends on the morale that gets passed down from above.

"The data suggest that good mental health retards midlife deterioration in physical health." This was the conclusion reached by George Vaillant, M.D., in his *New England Journal of Medicine* study. Male college sophomores with "no mental or physical problems" from the classes of

191

1942 to 1944 were selected as subjects. The 188 men underwent physical examinations and completed questionnaires at regular intervals, and Dr. Vaillant kept track of their mental and physical health over a period of thirty-two years. A clear pattern emerged.

Of the men who demonstrated the best mental health, only 3 percent became chronically ill or died by the age of fifty-three. In contrast, of those with the worst mental health, 38 percent became chronically ill or died. The effects of alcohol, cigarette smoking, obesity, and heredity were controlled statistically and did not influence results.

Our feelings are indeed powerful, and scientists more and more are beginning to understand why. Certain moods produce certain brain chemicals that in turn can affect the body in certain very specific ways, some good and some bad. Fear, for example, causes the release of adrenaline, which causes the heart to beat faster and blood flow to increase to the muscles in preparation for action. On an occasional basis this causes no problems, but if chronic, such as with the anxiety associated with a worrisome or distrustful view of the world, problems can arise. As we've mentioned earlier, chronic adrenaline flow can cause fat cells to release an excessive number of fat molecules into the blood, which in turn can cause the liver to increase its output of LDL cholesterol, the bad kind suspected of sticking to artery walls. Excess adrenaline also is suspected of damaging artery walls directly in a way that creates tiny "divots" capable of giving LDL cholesterol an even firmer footing.

Research shows that heart problems also can be worsened by loneliness and depression. The mechanisms by which these emotions do their damage are less clear, but the evidence is convincing, nonetheless. Depression proved in one group of heart disease patients to be a stronger predictor of future heart trouble than high cholesterol levels or smoking.

Then there's the immune system itself, that intricate network of chemical communication that protects us from everything from cancer to the common cold. Yes, genetic inheritance appears to play a strong role in a robust immune system, as we saw in chapter 5, but research leaves little doubt that immunity also is highly susceptible to changes in mental state. Positive feeling such as empathy, love, and even just a good laugh appear capable of boosting immunity (as measured by increases in germ-fighting cells in the saliva and blood) whereas negative emotions such as sadness, despair, and hate show evidence of diminishing the body's germ-fighting powers.

The effect that the mind can have over physical health has opened up a fascinating and very promising new field of medical research, and while a lot remains to be learned, an encouragingly simple message seems to be emerging: Enjoy life and you're likely to have more of it to enjoy. Happiness may be our most important nutrient of all. Maybe you've sensed this intuitively, and maybe you've witnessed it in relatives or friends. If you really love life, it takes a lot to take it away. Give a damn, however, and you give it up for grabs.

So what's our point here as we head into our concluding chapters?

Simply this: Any health endeavor is diminished by the degree to which it fails to satisfy the basic human RDA (recommended daily allowance) for peace of mind. Yes, try to be physically active and try to eat a nutritious low-fat diet, but do not give these endeavors priority over your more important needs for contentment and joy. Implement changes gradually and comfortably, "piece by peace," as we've said before. What sense does it make to live long, after all, if you're not enjoying the trip? Pursuing health in the wrong ways or for the wrong reasons, which some of us do, as you'll be seeing in these remaining chapters, can be as bad as not pursuing health at all. We need to be careful not to perfect the body at the expense of the soul. Don't follow the example of the marathon runner whose training begins to take precedence over personal relationships, or the gymnast whose vigilance against body fat begins to starve the very fun out of living.

We show respect for life by pursuing happiness as much as by pursuing physical health, but we show the most respect of all by pursuing both.

30

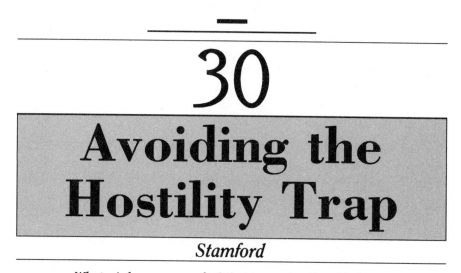

Avoiding the Hostility Trap

Stamford

What wisdom can you find that is greater than kindness?
—Jean-Jacques Rousseau, 1712–1778

The first time I met Ethan, I was intimidated. A successful business-man, obviously wealthy, distinguished-looking and charming—when he wanted to be. People at the cocktail party who "mattered" received a double dose of charm from Ethan, but those who didn't were ignored. I was content to be ignored, but a mutual acquaintance forced a quick first-name introduction, which lasted all of a few seconds.

I ran into Ethan in the park some weeks later. He had finished his run; mine was just beginning. He recognized me but reintroduced himself as if we had never met. "Mind if I tag along for a few more miles?" he said. "If this old body can keep up, that is." He positioned himself just in front of me, and we took off faster than I would have liked. As we ran, his pace quickened, faster and faster, until just short of the 3-mile mark I had to plead "uncle." Ethan stopped and walked back, grinning at my bent-over posture of defeat.

"I thought you were an exercise pro?" he scoffed. It was then that I realized what was going on. He knew, without my knowing it, who I was and what I did for a living. What's more, he was determined to beat me at what he thought was my own game. And he did.

I learned later that this was Ethan's approach to all aspects of life. Winning was everything, and he had to win at all costs. I haven't seen

194

Ethan since he added me to his trophy case, but newspaper accounts indicate he is still going at full throttle. From all outward appearances, he is healthy as a horse, but psychologically he is offering himself as a sitting duck.

"I think the mind is where heart disease starts for many people," says physician and heart specialist Dean Ornish, M.D., of the University of California at San Francisco. Dr. Ornish, as mentioned in chapter 4, has been directing a unique and very encouraging experiment since 1986. He has been trying to reverse the arterial blockage caused by heart disease by getting people to change their attitudes as well as their activity levels and eating habits.

His regimen includes walking and a very low-fat diet, but perhaps most importantly it includes daily classes designed to help people change their heart-damaging personalities. As of his report in 1989 at the sixty-first annual meeting of the American Heart Association, ten of his first twelve patients had experienced "meaningful overall reversal of their coronary atherosclerosis (blockage due to fatty buildup on artery walls)." They also experienced drops in their blood pressure and decreases in LDL cholesterol averaging 60 percent. These rates of improvement were in marked contrast to those of another group of people who had not taken part in Dr. Ornish's program but had received standard medical treatment, instead. Eleven of the seventeen patients in this group actually saw their arterial blockage get worse.

Had the low-fat diet and walking been the only reasons for the remarkable improvements in the Ornish group?

Dr. Ornish doesn't think so, and he has good reason not to. Considerable evidence has been accumulating since the 1950s suggesting that the mind's role in the heart disease process may be as important as the body's.

But wait a minute. Isn't stress as old as survival itself? And isn't adrenaline the high-octane fuel we relied on to get us through these times of extreme duress? If we had let the enraged beasts and famines and other calamities of nature get the best of us back then, we wouldn't still be here fighting the good fight today, correct?

Correct, except for one important difference: The good fight back then was either won or lost and that was the end of it. Either you got the beast or the beast got you. Not so today, when the beast may be a boss you'd like to see in a soup line, or a mortgage with a flexible interest rate that feels like it's strangling you.

Our stresses today tend to be less attackable, with the result being that we tend to feel endangered constantly. We feel we must continually be on guard because the "enemy"—our fellow man—is always out there. We feel we must be suspicious and basically mistrusting in order to survive, and yet the tragic irony is that it's our own survival that suffers in the process.

Researchers used to believe that any psychologically aggressive "Type A" behavior was a risk factor for heart disease, but in the past few years they've narrowed this view. Only aggressiveness that's rooted in hostility or mistrust appears to be dangerous. The go-getter who simply wants to go and get for the sake of prosperity appears to be off the hook. It's the people who want to go and get throats as much as money who appear to be at the greatest cardiovascular risk—the Ethans of the world.

Why?

Because to an evil eye, all looks evil. Mistrust creates an enemy whether there really is one or not. And with the mistrust, of course, comes the perpetual state of anxiety associated with having to be constantly on guard against this enemy. Whether the enemy is the electric company or the neighbor whose leaves won't seem to stay in his own yard, the mistrusting person suspects a motive, a larger plan that, like an iceberg, must be worried about and watched for at all times.

It's a bad way to navigate life. Research now leaves little doubt that a hostile and mistrusting attitude ranks right up there with extreme obesity, cigarette smoking, and a high-fat diet as a major risk factor for cardiovascular disease. Combine any of these factors and you've really got trouble.

Exercise and the Hostile Heart

And what sort of antidote might physical exercise be for the aggressive characteristics of a hostile heart?

All too often, unfortunately, strenuous physical exercise only gives hostile aggressions greater strength. People with deep-seated hostilities frequently reinforce their aggressions in their workouts by deriving energy from them. An old weight-lifting buddy of mine used to focus on his hatred for his former wife to give him energy for his heaviest lifts. Was this relieving him of his hostilities? Hardly. It was driving those hostilities even deeper into his mind with the force of whatever monstrous weight he was trying to lift.

As we mentioned back in chapter 7 in our discussion of exercise and stress, people who bring hostility to their exercise programs rarely sweat the hostility out. On the contrary, exercise seems only to give the hostility physical expression. As you may recall from that chapter, blood tests done on hostile/aggressive exercisers showed that they were not enjoying the same positive changes (as measured by increases in beneficial HDLs) as people who were exercising in a more relaxed and enjoyable manner. Being "out for blood" appeared not to be so good for the blood, with excess adrenaline being the suspected cause. The hostile/aggressive exerciser all too often comes away from a tough workout feeling more "pumped up" than "mellowed out."

Is this to suggest that a hostile attitude cannot be changed, that once a cynic always a cynic, destined to boil in one's own adrenal stew?

No, it just means that hard physical exercise is not a guaranteed cure, and that for some it can do more to feed the problem than fix it. Hostility is a psychological condition that needs to be remedied in a psychological way. Half the battle, moreover, may simply be wanting to change. Many hostile people enjoy the perch from which they cast their aspersions at the world because it feels safe. But safe it is not. It can be downright deadly, as we've seen. What scares the true cynic, ironically, is intimacy, because intimacy means dropping the defenses. Far easier and far safer to keep on guard, to expect and be prepared for the worst.

If any of this is ringing bells, you might be casting some aspersions of your own right now. Who are these softies? First they want you to lighten up in the weight room, and now they want you inviting the whole neighborhood over for tea.

That might not actually be a bad idea, eventually, but if you'd rather not take such a giant step at first, there are things you can do gradually and less dramatically to help sweeten a bitter heart.

Let's start with a little self-examination.

1. Do you find yourself placing blame on others when it doesn't belong? Do you, for example, feel like strangling the guy whose flat tire has caused you to get tied up in a thirty-minute traffic jam?

2. Do you perceive that you are always the intended victim? Is the woman in front of you in the express check-out lane purposely violating your rights by purchasing more items than she's allowed?

3. Do you tend not to speak out when you really should and then feel anger and even hatred toward those who are responsible for your discomfort?

4. Do you monopolize conversations by doing most of the talking?

5. Do you find yourself being cynical much of the time?

6. Do you hold grudges?

7. Do you feel that you have quick and simple answers to other people's problems? Others could manage their lives better, in other words, if they just saw the world as you do.

8. Do you always play to win, no matter what?

If you answered yes to more than one of these questions, you may have a hostile streak. Knowing it's there is a big step. Acknowledge it and pledge to work at being kinder to yourself by taking the following steps.

☐ *Instead of quickly placing blame on someone, place yourself in the other person's shoes.* Try to see things from his or her point of view. How would you feel if someone blamed you for something over which you have absolutely no control? Try to assume people have justifiable reasons for the way they behave and that their purpose in life is not merely to complicate yours.

☐ *Stop personalizing everything.* Chances are good that very few, if any, of the things that go wrong were intended for you personally. Things happen!

☐ *Learn to be constructively assertive.* Temper your anger with reason and control, and if something is wrong, say so in a way that dignifies your stance. A course in assertiveness training may help.

☐ *Learn to listen to what others are saying.* You can't gain perspective if you're the one who's always doing the talking. Hostile/aggressive people tend to be horrendous listeners, which only winds up feeding their self-centeredness. Make it a point to allow others to express themselves fully before you begin. Wait for lulls in conversation as your cue to start talking.

☐ Cynicism assumes that others are inferior, incompetent, or worse, and that they are not to be trusted. It's important whenever possible to *prove that assumption wrong.* If Johnny wants to take a shot at cutting the grass, give it to him. Even if you do have to remedy his effort, it shows you thought enough of him to give him the chance. You stand to benefit in the long run when you give people the benefit of the doubt. Give trust a trial run.

☐ Holding grudges is what holds hostility together, so it's important to *let ill feelings go.* Open the windows and let the stale air out. You and everyone else will breathe easier when you do.

☐ At the root of hostility is an attitude of selfishness, a feeling that the only person and the only opinion that really matters is one's own. *Try to keep a more open mind.*

☐ Winning isn't all it's cracked up to be. Take a look at all the times in your life that you've "won." Just exactly what did you win? Was it worth being hostile? Of course not. *Winning or losing has absolutely nothing to do with your value as a person.* Believe it and start living it.

☐ *Don't underestimate the power of positive thinking.* Replace negativism with positive thoughts and statements. Take time to convince yourself that the world is a pretty good place and that most of its inhabitants are pretty good folks. Look for the good things. Remember them and relate them to others.

☐ *Don't take yourself too seriously*. If you do, you'll be the only one who does. Look for life's little absurdities and laugh good-naturedly at them. Is it possible that the neighbor with the ill-behaved leaves really wants them in your yard, or that he wants your icy hellos at the mailbox? Ill will and a sense of humor have a very tough time getting along, so try to develop the latter.

In conclusion, may we say that life is short enough as it is. Why risk shortening it even more through mistrust? Research leaves little doubt that optimism and a positive view of the world relate closely to good physical health. Laboratory tests have shown that optimists tend to have stronger immune systems and that they recover from illnesses faster when they get sick. These studies would suggest that a mistrusting and hostile life attitude may in fact backfire, causing a kind of mutiny on a biological level against the person who holds such an attitude.

Don't risk it. Hostility is its own worst enemy. It's certainly no way to be victorious in the quest for long life. Got that, Ethan?

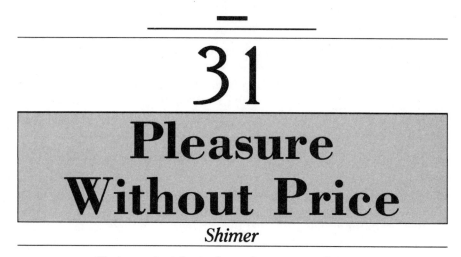

31

Pleasure Without Price

Shimer

That man is richest whose pleasures are cheapest.
—Henry David Thoreau, 1817–1862

Y ou're a long time dead, so why not enjoy life while you can?"

The man had a cigarette in one hand and a double scotch in the other, but he also had a point. If life is in fact finite, why not fill it with as much pleasure as possible, even if the consequence may be several fewer years? It's probably not much fun being ninety-five anyway.

We agree. We agree so totally, in fact, that we think pleasure should be sought on a level higher than just smoking or drinking. We suggest pursuit of the "mega-pleasure." (Please excuse the "popishness" of the term and to a degree the oversimplification it represents. Hopefully, the worth of our point will excuse this momentary breach of scientific standards.)

To understand the mega-pleasure you need first to understand pleasure in its lesser forms. Researchers now look at pleasure as existing on two levels: the physical and the mental. Physical pleasures are those that affect the senses directly—the sweet taste of an orange, the warmth of a hot bath, the smell of fresh flowers, the sound of pleasing music, or the sight of a beautiful landscape. Mental pleasures, on the other hand, involve the emotions—the joy felt at a graduation or wedding, the excitement experienced at a sporting event, the sense of accomplishment felt at the

200

conclusion of an important task, the love felt for another person. These pleasures soothe the soul more than the senses, but they are powerful experiences nonetheless.

And the mega-pleasure?

Simply a combination of the two, a pleasure that soothes the mind and the body all in one blissful stroke. If you can relish a meal for its nutritional value as much as its great taste, for example, you are experiencing a mega-pleasure. If you can enjoy a walk at sunset that allows you to relax and reflect, you are experiencing a mega-pleasure. If you can get a glow from a glass of wine before dinner as you think back on a rewarding day, you are experiencing a mega-pleasure. _The mega-pleasure is that which feels good in addition to being good for you_—one which satisfies emotionally as well as physically, one which makes sense in addition to catering to the senses.

The problem with many of our pleasures today, unfortunately, is that they tend to be heavy on the physical but light on the mental side. The barroom happy hour, for example, which may afford a blissful buzz but can give rise to negative feelings later in the form of a hangover mixed with pangs of guilt. The cigarette, which may relax or energize but cannot do so without also prompting feelings of worry about the health consequences. The large hot fudge sundae, which may be heaven going down but hell to think about in terms of calories. The cocaine, which is fun only until it's gone, along with a week's pay.

The greatest pleasures are those that hold up under intellectual scrutiny and last. The mega-pleasure goes beyond being just a treat and becomes a treasure, something to be savored later as well as at the moment—a great vacation, a great concert, or even just a great discussion. Some mega-pleasures even grow in value with the passage of time by providing fodder for soothing reflection.

It might even be argued that the scarcity of the mega-pleasure today is why we remain so pleasure "full" and yet so pleasure starved. We are reaching too often for pleasures that may satisfy physically but mentally create a pleasure drain. The result has been the unquenchable thirst for pleasure that many of us now feel. Consider, for example, the drinking spree that results in a hangover and guilt. More drinking is likely to ensue merely as a way of soothing those pains. Drug abuse follows the same course: Highs are followed by lows, which require more highs just for the user to feel he or she is breaking even. Even dietary abuses can be guilty of this sort of self-perpetuation. One hot fudge sundae can leave feelings of guilt or low-esteem, which may open the flood gates for two or three more as an attempt is made to drown those negative feelings with more of the pleasure that caused them in the first place. The dietary binge, like the alcoholic or drug binge, is an example of a physical pleasure being asked to provide the type of comfort that only a mental pleasure can give. And disaster, of course, is the result.

Might a solution simply be to reduce our quests for pleasure across the board, to become a little more Spartan and a little less Roman in our expectations of the amount of pleasure life should provide?

It might, but it's certainly not the best solution, because life *should* be highly pleasurable. Research leaves no doubt that pleasure and health are closely aligned, as we saw in our opening chapter to this section. When the human organism feels good, the message seems to get communicated to virtually every cell in the body. Studies show that the body's immune system, for example, can be bolstered by something as simple as a funny movie, a warm bath, or the caress of another person. Research also leaves little doubt that people who lead pleasurable and happy lives are significantly more resistant to heart disease and cancer. Possibly it all boils down to the will to live, a will that tends to be strongest, understandably, when life is most fun.

Mastering the Pleasure Scale

So how do we reach for the good pleasures and avoid the bad? How do we healthfully get the joy that we seem to need to function at our psychological as well as biological best?

It can help, first of all, to think of the human body as a scale of justice regarding pleasure. It has been programmed from the standpoint of basic survival to want to come out at least even when the pleasures of life are weighed against the pains. If the scale tips toward the side of pain, resentment and depression can develop. If the scale can be kept tilted slightly toward the side of pleasure, however, feelings of happiness, confidence, and a basic optimism about life will be the result. The problem with reaching too often for purely physical pleasure, however, is that the scale can land with a thud on the side of pain when the pleasure is over. The secret to a healthfully pleasurable life is to pursue pleasures that avoid that sort of crash.

But the secret also is to avoid experiencing too many of the pains that can motivate the search for such ill-fated pleasures in the first place—an unbearable although high-paying job, conflict with family members, or maybe just the pain of knowing you have your bad habit. When I was performing brutal workouts for an hour or more every day, part of the reason was the amount of wine I was drinking at night. The workouts were absolving me of the guilt. But when I eased up on the wine, I felt I could ease up on the workouts. Better yet, I no longer felt I needed the wine as compensation for the pain those workouts were causing me. I was able to put my scale of justice back into balance between weights of more sensible proportion.

The pain/pleasure trade-off is something to think about if you're currently under the spell of a bad habit you'd like to break. You may need to identify and reduce the pains in your life before you can begin effectively to reduce whatever pleasures you're using to balance those pains out.

But what if those pains are not obvious to you, or worse yet, are beyond your control such as with a job you need to keep for the security of your family?

That's a time for the mega-pleasure. These pleasures, remember, come 100 percent guilt-free. They please rationally as well as sensually. They are incapable of being abused. Dr. Stamford and I have put together a list of some pleasures we feel have potential for meeting the "mega" criteria but do not feel the list is in any way complete. Anything that feels good physically at the same time it satisfies emotionally or intellectually fills the bill. So be creative and come up with mega-pleasures of your own.

Following this list of suggested mega-pleasures, we have also come up with a formula for evaluating pleasure in general. Try applying the formula to what you consider to be the pleasurable aspects of your life. If you find that too many of your pleasures are coming up with low overall scores, you may have the answer to what may be your basic disgruntlement with life. You're pursuing pleasures that are really only pains in disguise.

Activities Capable of Mega-Pleasure Status

Heathful meals
Enjoyable exercise routine
Great vacations
Community service
Classes in art, music, or useful trade
Reading
Writing
Deepening communication, "connecting" with other people
A good movie
Sex
Gardening
Meaningful time with one's children
A good laugh
A good cry

Measure That Pleasure

For a pleasure to be truly pleasurable, it should satisfy mentally as well as physically. Any pleasure should be given penalty points, in fact, for the degree to which it causes uneasiness on the mental level.

So how do your pleasures measure up?

Rate them accordingly and find out: Assign the pleasure a number ranging from a +3 to a −3 in terms of how it satisfies physically, and then rate it in a similar fashion according to how it satisfies mentally. An apple, for example, might score only a +1 physically, but a +2 mentally because of its healthfulness. A cigarette, on the other hand, might score a +2 physically but a −3 mentally because of its unhealthfulness. So which is the greater pleasure?

Sorry, but our vote goes to the apple. We think you'll be surprised at the outcomes when you subject the pleasures in your own life to this test. Many of the little things we tend to take for granted are in fact our greatest pleasure of all when both their physical and mental contributions are considered. This may be why some of the happiest people can have such happiness despite appearing to have so little. They in truth have a great deal because their pleasures have so few negative aspects. Their pleasures allow them the greatest pleasure of all, which is a happy conscience. We include some other examples here of how various pleasures might be thought to stack up when all their ramifications are considered.

Note: Our pleasure formula is admittedly simplistic, and we in no way recommend that you carry around a note pad forever assigning numerical values to the joys in your life. To do so would be even more counterproductive to your overall goal of greater happiness than obsessing over a strict diet or a regimented exercise program. We offer this formula only to help make our point that not all pleasures are as supreme as they may seem, and that others are diamonds in the rough. The search for happiness, remember, is best aided by developing a taste for pleasures that come pain-free.

Activity	Physical Pleasure (ability to satisfy the senses)	Mental Pleasure (ability to satisfy the conscience)	Total
Inebriation at happy hour	+3	−2	+1
Glass of wine before dinner	+1	+2	+3
Coconut custard pie for dessert	+3	−1	+2
Piece of cantaloupe for dessert	+1	+3	+4

30-minute jog at 6:00 A.M.	0	+3	+3
30-minute walk at sunset	+2	+2	+4
Two hours high on drugs	+3	-3	0
Two hours at a stage play	+2	+2	+4
Smoking a cigarette	+3	-3	0
Taking a hot bath	+2	+2	+4
Driving a car that gets 14 mpg	+3	0	+3
Driving a car that gets 35 mpg	+1	+2	+3

A Word on Tolerance

Also important in maintaining a healthy relationship with pleasure is avoiding the tolerance trap. The body will begin to derive less effect from any substance the more the substance is used. The phenomenon is the body's way of striving to maintain "homeostasis," an internal order despite any disorder inflicted from outside. What homeostasis means for most pleasure-seekers, however, is nothing but trouble, as four drinks are eventually needed to do the job of one, or the cigarette that used to satisfy for several hours begins to satisfy only for several minutes.

Don't fall into the tolerance snare. If you choose not to quit a bad habit, at least cut down. You'll find yourself eventually getting far better "mileage" from your bad habit if you do.

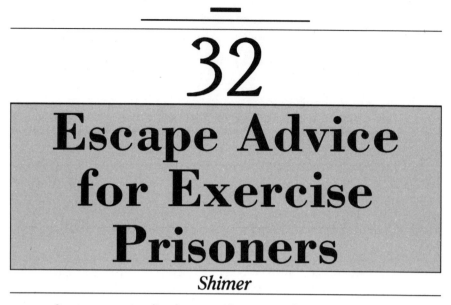

32

Escape Advice for Exercise Prisoners

Shimer

One can remain alive long . . . if one is unafraid of change. . . .
—Edith Wharton, 1862–1937

When Dr. Stamford asked me to tell the whole truth and nothing but the truth in this chapter, I had my reservations at first. Would it weaken our argument to confess the degree to which strenuous physical exercise has dominated my life?

We decided not. We decided it could only strengthen our argument by showing that strenuous exercise is not only unnecessary, but potentially highly addictive. I have exercised while ill and while injured. I have exercised in thunderstorms and blizzards. I have exercised instead of attending important functions with my family, and I have exercised my way out of more than one job.

Don't think this chapter is just about addiction to exercise, however. It's about addiction to regimentation in general. It's about being bound by routine and fear of change, and about the disservice we do ourselves by perpetuating the false sense of order that devotion to routine can provide. We tend to constrict and trivialize our lives in more ways than we realize, whether by needing to keep the pillows fluffed on the couch or being afraid to try a new brand of ketchup. We would rather feel secure in monotony than be challenged by change.

And yet in too much order there can be disorder. It might not give the appearance of disorder, but that's only because it's become so familiar.

Too much regimentation can prevent the kind of spontaneity and flexibility it takes to respond best to one's environment. Those of us bound to our routines miss out. We remain safe, but we often fail to capitalize on important opportunities in the process.

Keep these thoughts in mind as you hear my story. Whether you have an exercise problem or not, you might learn something. In re-evaluating my exercise habits, I found myself re-evaluating my life, and it's changed my life. A similar look at your own living patterns might help you. Where is your life bogging you down? Where's the drudgery and why? What are you gaining by remaining bound to your current routines? What might be passing you by because of those routines? Life's ruts can be dug by more than just a compulsion to jog the same path every day. You can work, eat, think, and drug your way into self-defeating consistency just as well.

So here we go. Yes, I went overboard with fitness, but in so doing I got a better look at the ship. The least I can do is help keep others from taking the same plunge.

The Blunder Years

When Dr. Stamford and I first began discussing this book, I was actually afraid the project might cure me. That's how dependent on my workouts I was. I counted on them for self-esteem, a sense of order and control, a feeling of accomplishment, an element of hardship, a hefty drinking habit, a way to annoy my mother-in-law, a form of punishment.

It was a strange brew of benefits, as you can see, and not all of them positive. That realization alone was extremely helpful for me. I used to think there was something almost holy about the pain and exhaustion of a tortuous workout, but it gradually occurred to me that devilish might actually be the better word. Any sort of purification I used to feel from those killer workouts was only allowing my "pollutions" to continue. With alcohol, for example, I'd feel that a really tough workout deserved to be rewarded that night with a few extra drinks, only to feel obligated to work out that much harder the next day as punishment for the overindulgence. But then the hard workout would only set me up for another reward, and the spiral would continue. Not only was it an absurd cycle, but an exhausting one.

How had exercise entered my life in the first place, and at what point did it start to overpower me?

I was precocious—at least I can say that. I was overdosing on exercise by the time I was thirteen. I used to put paper towels between the plates of the barbells so my two older brothers wouldn't hear me doing bench presses at 10:30 at night in the basement. The sound used to travel up through the heating ducts all the way to our bedroom in the attic. I even had to be careful not to grunt too loud. My brothers had no sympathy for my efforts because they were already strong. They looked at lifting weights as an admission of weakness. My oldest brother could lift the front end of a Volkswagen beetle off the ground by the time he was seventeen. He was six feet tall and weighed 180 pounds by the time he was in the eighth grade. He was so big in Little League that he had to wear a special uniform from an adult softball league.

I learned later that Bob suffered from being so large, but that didn't make his belittling me any easier. I wouldn't stand for it, though. We laugh about it now, but we'd get into fights that lasted an entire day. He'd beat me up once, politely but nonetheless decidedly, and I'd slink off to recuperate. An hour or so later I'd come at him again, ambush-style this time, from a doorway or bush, and there'd be another sound thrashing. Strike three could come as late as that night after dinner, but not until then would I count myself "out." Twenty years later I'd be using that same kind of stupidity to run a 3:15 marathon on my first try.

Brother number two was different. He didn't have Bob's size, but he had the kind of speed and coordination that made size irrelevant. Our scrapes would be ugly enough for me to learn not to scrape Andy very often.

So what's the point? Why the family history here?

Behind the exercise addiction is a reason for exercising that at one point might have made some sense. For me it was trying to keep pace with two very physical older brothers. But at some point the exercise becomes divorced from that initial sense of reason and becomes something else. It becomes a sanctuary, a place where the exerciser can feel both powerful and safe because he or she finally feels in control. Whether or not the initial reason for exercising has been satisfied doesn't matter—I still can't beat up either of my brothers—but the exercise provides comfort nonetheless. This isn't to say the exercise is approached in a relaxed manner, because often it is made to be very grueling, but there is comfort in the pain because at least its rules and its limits are in the hands of the exerciser. No more "big brothers" to dictate the score. The exerciser can batter himself.

But the sad irony, of course, is that the exerciser is not in control, because he or she is totally dominated by his or her habit. Even that sense of being dominated gives a feeling of security, however, because it eliminates choice. The enslavement to exercise precludes any need for having to make a decision whether or not to do it. The exerciser will exercise come hell or high water, and for more than a decade—ending in 1989—

I missed only one day of exercise, and not because of illness. I was on a series of plane flights that lasted sixteen hours, and even then I managed to squeeze in more isometrics than my seat partner would have liked.

How could any thinking person rationalize such a streak?

The streak, of course, became part of the problem. The longer it went on the more afraid I was to break it. An element of superstition begins to enter into any routine if it goes on long enough, even if it's just in the way you make your bed.

The bed I was making, however, was getting progressively tougher to lie in because I was making my workouts progressively tougher to do. And that's where the trap began to come down around me. It's the danger zone for all regular exercisers and research shows why. The amount of endorphins (mood-elevating chemicals) that strenuous exercise produces begins to diminish as you get in shape, the result being that you need to escalate your workouts either in length or intensity to get the same good feelings that might have come relatively easily early on. It's a phenomenon all regular exercisers need to be aware of to keep from being lured into the addiction snare. If you find you're no longer getting your customary "high" from your workouts, cut back or take some time off. Do *not* escalate your workouts. You'll wind up as I did if you do—like a donkey chasing a carrot at the end of a stick.

Going Cool Turkey

So what finally awakened me to my folly? Did I have a spill on the ice while jogging, like Dr. Stamford, or a severe injury that forced me out of my rut?

Sometimes I'd actually wish for such an injury, something to break the cycle for me, something that would force me to relinquish the very control that I had worked so hard to attain. After nearly thirty years I was finally sick to death of it. I wanted freedom from my own ridiculous set of rules. It's not that I was ready to give up to the point of becoming an overnight lush, but did I really need to be able to run a sub-three-hour marathon at the drop of a hat? Or to be able to wash my t-shirt on my stomach muscles when I took my shower?

And that's when I started to see a glimmer of hope. It was all simply a matter of degree. Exercise wasn't killing me, it was the amount that was killing me. As Dr. Stamford and I started working through the research for this book, it became clear to me that I was doing approximately four times as much exercise as I needed to for good health. And why? So that I could feel better about playing rough house with my liver with a liter of wine at night? Or feel guilty about not having enough time for my family? Or see the worried look on my mother-in-law's face when I'd come in from a 10-mile run in my rubber sweat suit and Navy pea coat in mid-June? What was I trying to prove? And to whom?

The abuse finally had to stop. Not all at once, perhaps—I knew myself better than that. But just as I had gotten myself into this mess gradually, I could get myself out of it gradually. I decided that by cutting back by just a few minutes a day, I could eventually be exercising "normally" and hopefully not suffer any great physical or psychological repercussions along the way. I had to start looking at less as being more.

And has it worked?

I've relapsed occasionally, but my overall progress has been excellent. I'm even now doing household chores in the place of workouts sometimes, as we recommend in this book, and that's felt like my greatest victory of all. I've also been surprised at how tough some of those chores can be. I used to scoff when green thumb types would tell me what great exercise gardening can be, but having a 20- by 40-foot patch of my own now, and no Rototiller, I've changed my thinking. I'm also doing some light weight training once or twice a week, on Dr. Stamford's advice, and that's helped me appreciate the value of variety. I've even learned to take days off entirely and to view it as a show of strength rather than weakness when I do.

So whether you're compulsive about exercise, your career, or even just having to have the cap on the toothpaste before you can go to bed at night, do yourself the favor of thinking about the larger scheme of things. Take off the blinders. Have the intelligence and good sense to consider the long-term value of your actions. As Dr. Stamford said back at the close of our opening section, at some point we need to step off our treadmills if we're ever going to find where our energies are really capable of taking us. I stepped off my treadmill and I feel like Hercules unchained. I didn't realize how much energy I was pouring into my exercise enslavement. I still have a way to go before I'm where I want to be, but at least I'm no longer just running in place.

Thoughts for the Enslaved

The following notions were helpful to me in making my exercise escape. Try them on for size. You may find them useful for overthrowing more than just a tyrannical commitment to fitness.

☐ *Realize that flexibility can be more valuable than strength.* Rigid self-discipline can serve a specific endeavor to which it's applied, but it also can hinder the kind of imagination and adaptability required for growth. Learn to bend, in other words, and you'll be less likely to break.

☐ *Stop trying to make every day perfect.* Like a good painting or a good song, variety of texture and mood, not a continuum of identical pieces, is what makes a work of art. Learn to accept life's lulls, and its crescendoes will only be that much more uplifting.

☐ *Respect the value of rest.* As former marathon champion Bill Rodgers once told me, "I've learned to look at missed workouts as being able to help me more than hurt me." Wise words. Even the best of batteries needs occasionally to be recharged.

☐ *Don't let today's accomplishment become tomorrow's obligation.* This means learning to enjoy high points without feeling they must be immediately duplicated or surpassed. Progress and success are better savored than gulped.

☐ *Look at missed workouts as victories rather than defeats.* They're a sign that you're showing the confidence to break free of your routine. Find something constructive to do with that energy and you've really got something to celebrate.

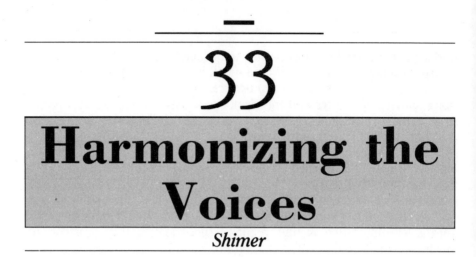

33

Harmonizing the Voices

Shimer

Fortunately [psycho]analysis is not the only way to resolve inner conflicts. Life itself still remains a very effective therapist.
—Karen Horney, 1885–1952

I was staring into a blank sheet of paper trying to come up with a good way to introduce our concluding message for this book when inspiration came by way of an unlikely source. I could overhear the TV in the room next door, where my seven-year-old was watching cartoons, and there was Daffy Duck, as usual being torn between his devilish and angelic sides. His devilish side was exhorting him to do the unspeakable while his heavenly half was demanding he behave.

Millions of us in our pursuit of fitness, unfortunately, have found ourselves similarly torn. We've been hearing two voices, one telling us that the cheesecake in the refrigerator has our name on it, the other reminding us of its calories; the one saying, "Workout on the exercise bike," the other saying, "Stretch out on the couch."

Until a closer harmony can be achieved between these two voices, our goals for greater fitness and health are going to remain impossible dreams. We need to make our health and fitness efforts more intrinsically satisfying so that these two voices can become essentially one.

This became clear to me in a recent discussion I had with a friend who has been trying desperately to lose weight. "One voice says go ahead and break the diet because life's too short," she said. "But the other says

212

no, endure the pain because you've got a long way to go and you've got to make up for lost time."

That sense of urgency has been our health and fitness downfall. There is no making up for lost time, there is only making the best of current time. Too often we embark on regimens thinking that short-term pain is going to produce long-term success. But the body objects very strongly to working that way. Biological adaptation, whether it's toward weight loss or greater fitness, takes time. The body prefers to be coaxed rather than kicked, and the sooner those of us attempting health kicks realize that, the better.

Dr. Stamford, as you'll recall, has what he calls his "80/20 rule," and it's a good one. He tries to be "good" 80 percent of the time and doesn't worry about the 20 percent of the time he's "bad." This allows a vent for the very natural and very healthy need for occasional sprees, be they dietary or physical, such as in the form of a Sunday spent lifting nothing heavier than the Sunday paper. Too many of us attempt health regimes with no such "pit stops" for refueling. Instead we try to be perfect from start to finish, the result being that we either run out of steam short of our goals or find ourselves on dead empty at the finish. Any health effort has to be mindful of what lies ahead once the "race" is over. Is the crash dieter going to be able to subsist on liquid protein once weight-loss goals have been met? Is the maniacal iron-pumper going to be able to sustain his or her efforts gracefully into middle age?

Very unlikely. We need to gauge our health efforts so that they can nourish us rather than exhaust us. The past twenty years have been less of a fitness boom than a fitness battle, and overzealousness has been the reason. Nine out of ten diets have failed and eight out of ten fitness efforts have failed not because we haven't tried, but because we've tried too hard. We need to slow down, to relax, to allow our biology the time it needs to feel comfortable with the changes we're trying to make. Only that way can the discord between our two voices be resolved. As my overweight friend said, "It's as though my mind wants one thing and my body wants another."

That's the conflict we need to resolve. We have to get mind and body wanting the same thing. Nutritionally it can be done by eating delicious, yet low-fat and low-calorie meals. And if and when the body does express desire for a splurge, we should comply, guilt-free. Harmony on the exercise front can be achieved in a similar fashion. We shouldn't even put our bodies in the position of having to cry "uncle." Pain and boredom can be avoided by getting "workouts" in ways that are practical or fun.

"Piece by peace." We've said it before, but we'll say it again. There can be no lasting health that exists on conflict. And there are no short-term solutions for long-term goals. If that disappoints the impatience in you, so be it. We should enjoy the journey we make toward better health or perhaps not make it.

But can such a casual approach to better health really work?

It's the only way it can work because it's the only way it can last. Keep this in mind when working toward the specific goals we have given you in this book. The numbers can appear intimidating—2,000 calories of activity a week and a 20 percent fat diet based on no more than 45 grams of fat a day. Consider these numbers to be long-term goals rather than immediate obligations, and don't feel bad if you never achieve them at all. Any progress you make is better than no progress. Your goal should be to improve your health, but not at the expense of your happiness. Good luck.

References

Part I

Allison, T. G., R. M. Iammarino, K. F. Metz, *et al.* "Failure of Exercise to Increase High Density Lipoprotein Cholesterol." *Journal of Cardiac Rehabilitation* 1:257–265, 1981.

American College of Sports Medicine position statement: "The Recommended Quality and Quantity of Exercise for Developing and Maintaining Fitness in Healthy Adults." *Sports Medicine Bulletin* 13:1, 1978.

American Heart Association. *1988 Heart Facts*. National Center, Dallas, Texas.

Amodeo, C., and F. H. Messerli. "Risk for Obesity." *Cardiology Clinics* 4:75–80, 1986.

Astrand, P. O. "From Exercise Physiology to Preventive Medicine." *Annals of Clinical Research* 20:10–17, 1988.

Barrett-Connor, E. L. "Obesity, Atherosclerosis and Coronary Heart Disease." *Annals of Internal Medicine* 103:1010–1019, 1985.

Bassler, T. J. Letter. *Lancet* 2:711–712, 1972.

Biss, K., K. J. Ho, B. Mikkelson, *et al.* "Some Unique Biologic Characteristics of the Masai of East Africa." *New England Journal of Medicine* 284:694–699, 1971.

Blackburn, H. "Physical Activity and Coronary Heart Disease: A Brief Update and Population View" (Part I). *Journal of Cardiac Rehabilitation* 3:101–111, 1983.

Blair, S. N., and H. W. Kohl, R. S. Paffenbarger, *et al.* "Physical Fitness and All-Cause Mortality: A Prospective Study of Healthy Men and Women." *Journal of the American Medical Association* 262:2395–2401, 1989.

Blair, S. N. "Physical Activity Leads to Fitness and Pays Off." *The Physician and Sportsmedicine* 13(3):153–157, 1985.

Blair, S. N., K. H. Cooper, L. W. Gibbons, *et al.* "Changes in Coronary Heart

Disease Risk Factors Associated with Increased Treadmill Time in 753 Men." *American Journal of Epidemiology* 118(Sept.):352–359, 1983.

Breslow, L., and P. Buell. "Mortality from Coronary Heart Disease and Physical Activity of Work in California." *Journal of Chronic Disease* 11:421–444, 1960.

Brooks, C. "Adult Physical Activity Behavior: A Trend Analysis." *Journal of Clinical Epidemiology* 41(4):385–392, 1988.

Brooks, C. "Adult Participation in Physical Activities Requiring Moderate to High Levels of Energy Expenditure." *The Physician and Sportsmedicine* 15(4):119–132, 1987.

Brownell, K. D., P. S. Bachorik, and R. S. Ayerle. "Changes in Plasma Lipid and Lipoproteins Levels in Men and Women After a Program of Moderate Exercise." *Circulation* 65:477–483, 1982.

Brunner, D., G. Manelis, M. Modan, *et al.* "Physical Activity at Work and the Incidence of Myocardial Infarction, Angina Pectoris and Death Due to Ischemic Heart Disease: An Epidemiological Study in Israeli Collective Settlements (Kibbutzim)." *Journal of Chronic Disease* 27:217–233, 1974.

Caspersen, C., and R. A. Pollard. "Prevalence of Physical Activity in the United States and Its Relationship to Disease Risk Factors." *Medicine and Science in Sports and Exercise* 19(2):31, 1987 (abstract).

Cassel, J., S. Heyden, A. G. Barte, *et al.* "Occupation and Physical Activity and Coronary Heart Disease." *Archives of Internal Medicine* 128:920–928, 1971.

Connor, W. E., M. T. Cerquera, T. W. Connor, *et al.* "The Plasma Lipids, Lipoproteins and Diet of the Tarahumara Indians of Mexico." *American Journal of Clinical Nutrition* 31:1131–1142, 1978.

Constant, J. "Nutritional Management of Diet-Induced Hyperlipidemias and Atherosclerosis: Part III." *Internal Medicine* 8:95–103, 1987.

Cook, T. C., R. E. LaPorte, R. A. Washburn, *et al.* "Chronic Low Level Physical Activity as a Determinant of High Density Lipoprotein Cholesterol and Subfractions." *Medicine and Science in Sports and Exercise* 18(6):653–657, 1986.

Cooper, K. H., M. L. Pollock, R. P. Martin, *et al.* "Physical Fitness Levels vs. Selected Coronary Risk Factors: A Cross-Sectional Study." *Journal of American Medical Association* 236(Jul. 12):166–169, 1976.

Cooper, K. H. *Aerobics.* New York, NY: Bantam Books, 1968.

Ehnolm, C., J. K. Huttunen, P. Pietinen, *et al.* "Effect of Diet on Serum Lipoproteins in a Population with a High Risk of Coronary Heart Disease." *New England Journal of Medicine* 307:850–855, 1982.

Ekelund, L., W. L. Haskell, J. L. Johnson, *et al.* "Physical Fitness as a Predictor of Cardiovascular Mortality in Asymptomatic North American Men." *New England Journal of Medicine* 319:1379–1384, 1988.

Enos, W. F., R. H. Holmes, and J. Beyer. "Coronary Disease Among United States Soldiers Killed in Korea." *Journal of American Medical Association* 152:1090–1093, 1953.

Executive Fitness Newsletter. "Are You a 'Type A' Exerciser?" 18(9):1–2, 1987.

Frank, C. W., E. Weinblatt, S. Shapiro, *et al.* "Myocardial Infarction in Men." *Journal of American Medical Association* 198(12):1241–1245, 1966.

Froilicher, V. F. "Exercise and the Prevention of Coronary Atherosclerotic Heart Disease." In Wenger, N. K. (ed.), *Exercise and the Heart.* Philadelphia: F. A. Davis Co., 1978, pp. 13–23.

Gibbons, L. W., S. N. Blair, K. H. Cooper, *et al.* "Association Between Coronary Heart Disease Risk Factors and Physical Fitness in Healthy Adult Women." *Circulation* 67(May):977–983, 1983.

Gordon, D. J., J. Knoke, J. L. Probstfield, *et al.* "High-Density Lipoprotein Cholesterol and Coronary Heart Disease in Hypercholesterolemic Men: The Lipid Research Clinics Primary Prevention Trial." *Circulation* 74:1217–1225, 1986.

Greist J. H., M. H. Klein, R. R. Eischens, *et al.* "Running as Treatment for Depression." *Compr. Psychiatry* 20(Jan.–Feb.):41–54, 1979.

Griffin, G. C., and W. P. Castelli. "All About Your Cholesterol Numbers." *Prevention* 55–59, March 1989.

Grundy, M. S. "Monounsaturated Fatty Acids Plasma Cholesterol, and Coronary Heart Disease." *American Journal of Clinical Nutrition* 45:1237–1242, 1987.

Haskell, W. L. "Physical Activity and Health: Need to Define the Required Stimulus." *American Journal of Cardiology* 5:4D–9D, 1985.

Herbert, P. N., D. N. Bernier, E. M. Cullinane, *et al.* "High-density Lipoprotein Metabolism in Runners and Sedentary Men." *Journal of American Medical Association* 252:1034–1037, 1984.

Heyden, S., and G. J. Fodor. "Does Regular Exercise Prolong Life Expectancy?" *Sports Medicine* 6:63–71, 1988.

Holman, R. L., H. C. McGill, Jr., J. P. Strong, *et al.* "The Natural History of Atherosclerosis." *American Journal of Pathology* 34:209–235, 1958.

Huttunen, J. K., E. Lansimies, E. Voutilainen, *et al.* "Effect of Moderate Physical Exercise on Serum Lipoproteins: A Controlled Clinical Trial with Special Reference to Serum High Density Lipoproteins." *Circulation* 60:1220–1229, 1979.

International Collaborative Group. "Circulating Cholesterol Level and Risk of Death from Cancer in Men Aged 40–69 Years—Experience of International Collaborative Group." *Journal of American Medical Association* 248:2853–2859, 1982.

Jacoby, D. B. "Physical Activity and Longevity of College Alumni" (letter). *New England Journal of Medicine* 315(6):399, 1986.

Kahn, H. A. "The Relationship of Reported Coronary Heart Disease Mortality to Physical Activity of Work." *American Journal of Public Health* 53:1058–1067, 1963.

Kaplan, N. M., and J. Stamler. *Prevention of Coronary Heart Disease: Practical Management of the Risk Factors*. Philadelphia: W. B. Saunders Company, 1983.

Kark, J. D., A. H. Smith, and C. G. Hames. "The Relationship of Serum Cholesterol to the Incidence of Cancer in Evans County, Georgia." *Journal of Chronic Disease* 33:311–322, 1980.

Keys, A., A. Menotti, M. J. Karvonen, *et al*. "The Diet and 15-Year Death Rate in the Seven Countries Study." *American Journal of Epidemiology* 124:403–415, 1986.

Kowalski, R. E. *The 8-Week Cholesterol Cure*. New York: Harper & Row, Publishers, 1987.

LaPorte, R., and D. LaPorte. "A New Look at Exercise and Fitness." *Executive Health Report* XXIV(12):1–2, 1988.

LaPorte, R. E., S. Dearwater, J. A. Cauley, *et al*. "Physical Activity or Cardiovascular Fitness: Which Is More Important for Health? *The Physician and Sportsmedicine* 13:145–150, 1985.

LaPorte, R. E., L. L. Adams, D. D. Savage, *et al*. "The Spectrum of Physical Activity, Cardiovascular Disease and Health: An Epidemiological Perspective." *American Journal of Epidemiology* 120:507–517, 1984.

Legwold, G. "Are We Running from the Truth About the Risks and Benefits of Exercise?" *The Physician and Sportsmedicine* 13(5):136–148, 1985.

Leon, A. S. (letter). *Journal of American Medical Association* 259(9):1328, 1988.

Leon, A. S., J. Connett, D. R. Jacobs, *et al*. "Leisure-Time Physical Activity Levels and Risk of Coronary Heart Disease and Death." *Journal of American Medical Association* 258:2388–2395, 1987.

Leon, A. S., and H. Blackburn. "Physical Activity in the Prevention of Coronary Heart Disease: An Update 1981." In C. B. Arnold (ed.). *Advances in Disease Prevention*. Vol. 1. New York: Springer Publishing Co., pp. 97–133, 1981.

Leon, A. S., J. Conrad, D. B. Hunninghake, *et al*. "Effects of a Vigorous Walking Program on Body Composition, and Carbohydrate and Lipid Metabolism of Obese Young Men." *American Journal of Clinical Nutrition* 32:1776–1787, 1979.

Levy, R. I. "Consideration of Cholesterol and Noncardiovascular Mortality." *American Heart Journal* 104:324–328, 1982.

Lipid Research Clinic Program. "The Lipid Research Clinics Coronary Primary Prevention Trial II. The Relationship of Reduction in Incidence of Coronary Heart Disease to Cholesterol Lowering." *Journal of American Medical Association* 251:365–374, 1984.

Magnus, R., A. Matroos, and J. Stracklee. "Walking, Cycling, or Gardening with or Without Season Interruption in Relation to Acute Coronary Events. *American Journal of Epidemiology* 110:724–33, 1979.

Mahley, R. W. "The Role of Dietary Fat and Cholesterol in Atherosclerosis and Lipoprotein Metabolism." *Western Journal of Medicine* 134:34–42, 1981.

Mann, G. V., R. D. Shaffer, R. S. Anderson, *et al.* "Cardiovascular Disease in the Masai." *Journal of Atherosclerosis Research* 4:289–312, 1964.

McNamara, J. J., M. A. Molot, J. F. Stremple, *et al.* "Coronary Artery Disease in Combat Casualties in Vietnam." *Journal of American Medical Association* 216:1185–1187, 1971.

Menotti, A., V. Puddu, M. Monti, *et al.* "Habitual Physical Activity and Myocardial Infarction." *Cardiologia* 54:119–128, 1969.

Miettinen, T. A. "Dietary Fiber and Lipids." *American Journal of Clinical Nutrition* 45:1237–1242, 1987.

Moll, M. E., R. S. Williams, R. M. Lester, *et al.* "Cholesterol Metabolism in Non-Obese Women: Failure of Physical Conditioning to Alter Levels of High Density Lipoprotein Cholesterol. *Atherosclerosis* 34:159–166, 1979.

Monahan, T. "From Activity to Eternity." *The Physician and Sportsmedicine* 14:161, 1986.

Moncada, S., and J. R. Vance. "Arachidonic Acid Metabolites and the Interactions Between Platelets and Blood-vessel Walls." *New England Journal of Medicine* 300:1142–1147, 1979.

Morgan, W. P., and S. E. Goldston (eds.). *Exercise and Mental Health,* Washington, DC: Hemisphere Publishing, 1987.

Morris, J. N., J. A. Heady, P. A. Raffle, *et al.* "Coronary Heart Disease and Physical Activity of Work." *Lancet* 2:1053–1057, 1953.

Nestel, P. J., T. Billington, and B. Smith. "Low Density and High Density Lipoprotein Kinetics and Sterol Balance in Vegetarians." *Metabolism* 30:941–945, 1981.

Noakes, T. D., L. H. Opie, A. G. Rose. "Marathon Running and Immunity to Coronary Heart Disease: Fact Versus Fiction," in Franklin, B. A., and M. Rubenfire (eds): *Clinics in Sports Medicine* 3:527–543, 1984.

Oldridge, N. B. "Compliance and Exercise in Primary and Secondary Prevention of Coronary Heart Disease: A Review." *Preventive Medicine* 11:56–70, 1982.

Olsen, E. "Putting Fun Back in Fitness." *Reader's Digest*, pp. 145–150, August 1988.

Paffenbarger, R. S., Jr., R. T. Hyde, A. L. Wing, *et al*. "Physical Activity, All-Cause Mortality, and Longevity of College Alumni." *New England Journal of Medicine* 314:605–613, 1986.

Paffenbarger, R. S., Jr., and R. T. Hyde. "Exercise in the Prevention of Coronary Heart Disease." *Preventive Medicine* 13:3–22, 1984.

Paffenbarger, R. S., Jr., A. L. Wing, R. T. Hyde. "Physical Activity as an Index of Heart Attack Risk in College Alumni." *American Journal of Epidemiology* 108:161–175, 1978.

Paffenbarger, R. S., Jr., and W. E. Hale. "Work Activity and Coronary Heart Mortality." *New England Journal of Medicine* 292:545–550, 1975.

Paffenbarger, R.S., Jr., M. E. Laughlin, A. S. Gima, *et al*. "Work Activity of Longshoremen as Related to Death from Coronary Heart Disease and Stroke." *New England Journal of Medicine* 282:1109–1114, 1970.

Peters, R. K., L. D. Cady, Jr., D. P. Bischoff, *et al*. "Physical Fitness and Subsequent Myocardial Infarction in Healthy Workers." *Journal of American Medical Association* 249(22):3052–3056, 1983.

Petty, B. G., and D. M. Herrington. "Physical Activity and Longevity of College Alumni" (letter). *New England Journal of Medicine* 315(6):399, 1986.

Physician and Sportsmedicine. "The Health Benefits of Exercise" (Part 2 of 2) 15(11):121–131, 1987.

Pine, D. "Study Links Low Fitness Levels with CHD Deaths." *The Physician and Sportsmedicine* 17(1):42–43, 1989.

Ramlow, J., A. Kriska, and R. LaPorte. "Physical Activity in the Population: The Epidemiologic Spectrum." *Research Quarterly for Exercise and Sport* 58(2):11–114, 1987.

Rauramaa, R., J. T. Salonen, K. Kukkonen-Harjula, *et al*. "Effects of Mild Physical Exercise on Serum Lipoproteins and Metabolites of Arachidonic Acid: A Controlled Randomised Trial in Middle-Aged Men." *British Medical Journal* 288:603–606, 1984.

Saturday Evening Post. "High Cholesterol in Children." April 1989, pp. 42–43.

Schlierf, G., A. Lenore, P. Oster. "Influence of Diet on High-density Lipoproteins." *American Journal of Cardiology* 52:17B–19B, 1983.

Schmidt, J. E. "Jogging May Be Hazardous to Your Health." *The Louisville Times*, May 10, 1975.

Schaefer, O. "Vigorous Exercise and Coronary Heart Disease." *Lancet* I.840, 1973.

Schindler, J. *How to Live 365 Days a Year*. Greenwich, Conn.: Fawcett, Publishers, 1970.

Schucker, B. "Change in Public Perspective on Cholesterol and Heart Disease: Results from Two National Surveys." *Journal of American Medical Association* 258:3527–3531, 1987.

Siscovick, D. S., L. G. Ekelund, J. S. Hyde, *et al.* "Physical Activity and Coronary Heart Disease Among Asymptomatic Hypercholesterolemic Men." *American Journal of Public Health* 78(11):1428–1431, 1989.

Solomon, H. A. *The Exercise Myth*, New York: Harcourt, Brace, Jovanovich, Publishers, 1984.

Sopko, G., D. R. Jacobs, Jr., R. Jeffery, *et al.* "Effects on Blood Lipids and Body Weight in High Risk Men of a Practical Exercise Program. *Atherosclerosis* 49:219–229, 1983.

Sorensen, T. I. A., G. G. Nielsen, P. K. Andersen, *et al.* "Genetic and Environmental Influences on Premature Death in Adult Adoptees." *New England Journal of Medicine* 318:727–732, 1988.

"Sports Medicine: Where Do We Go from Here?" *The Physician and Sportsmedicine* 16:176, 1988.

Stamford, B. A., S. Matter, R. D. Fell, *et al.* "Cigarette Smoking, Physical Activity, and Alcohol: Relationship to Blood Lipids and Lipoproteins in Pre-menopausal Females. *Metabolism* 23:585–590, 1984.

Stamford, B. A., S. Matter, R. D. Fell, *et al.* "Cigarette Smoking, Exercise and High-Density Lipoprotein Cholesterol. *Atherosclerosis* 52:73–83, 1984.

Stephens, T., D. R. Jacobs, and C. C. White. "The Descriptive Epidemiology of Leisure-Time Physical Activity." *Public Health Report* 100:147–158, 1985.

Sutherland, W. H. F., and S. P. Woodhouse. "Physical Activity and Plasma Lipoprotein Lipid Concentrations in Men." *Atherosclerosis* 37:285–292, 1980.

Taylor, H. L., E. Klepetar, A. Keys, *et al.* "Death Rates Among Physically Active and Sedentary Employees of the Railroad Industry." *American Journal of Public Health* 52:1697–1707, 1962.

Thompson, P. D., E. M. Cullinane, S. P. Sady, *et al.* "Modest Changes in High-Density Lipoprotein Concentration and Metabolism with Prolonged Exercise Training." *Circulation* 78 (1):25–34, 1988.

Thompson, P. D., B. Lazarus, E. Cullinane, *et al.* "Exercise, Diet or Physical Characteristics as Determinants of HDL Levels in Endurance Athletes." *Atherosclerosis* 46:333–339, 1983.

Tuomilehto, J., B. Marti, J. T. Salonen, *et al.* "Leisure-Time Physical Activity Is Inversely Related to Risk Factors for Coronary Heart Disease in Middle-Aged Finnish Men." *European Heart Journal* 8:1047–1055, 1987.

Ulene, A. *Count Out Cholesterol*. New York: Feeling Fine Programs, Inc., and Alfred A. Knopf, Inc., 1989.

U.S. Department of Health and Human Services, Public Health Service: *Promoting Health and Preventing Disease: Objectives for the Nation.* Washington, D.C.: Supt. of Documents, U.S. Government Printing Office, Fall 1980.

Waller, B. F. "Exercise-Related Sudden Death." *Postgraduate Medicine* 83(8):273–282, 1988.

Waller, B. F. "Sudden Death in Middle-aged Conditioned Subjects; Coronary Atherosclerosis Is the Culprit." *Mayo Clinic Proceedings* 62(7):634–636, 1987.

Waller, B. F. "Exercise-Related Sudden Death in Young (Age <30 Years) and Old (Age >30 Years) Conditioned Subjects." *Cardiovascular Clinics* 15(2):9–73, 1985.

Waller, B. F., and W. C. Roberts. "Sudden Death While Running in Conditioned Runners Aged 40 Years or Over." *American Journal of Cardiology* 45(6):1292–300, 1980.

Weltman, A., S. Matter, and B. A. Stamford. "Caloric Restriction and/or Mild Exercise: Effects on Serum Lipids and Body Composition." *American Journal of Clinical Nutrition* 33:1002–1009, 1980.

Williams, P. I., P. D. Wood, W. L. Haskell, *et al.* "The Effects of Running Mileage and Duration on Plasma Lipoprotein Levels." *Journal of American Medical Association* 247:2674–9, 1982.

Williams, R. R. "Nature, Nurture and Family Disposition." (editorial). *New England Journal of Medicine* 318:769–771, 1988.

Williams, R. R., S. J. Hasstedt, D. E. Wilson, *et al.* "Evidence That Men with Familial Hypercholesterolemia Can Avoid Early Coronary Death: An Analysis of 77 Gene Carriers in Four Utah Pedigrees."*Journal of American Medical Association* 255:219–224, 1986.

Wood, P. D., W. L. Haskell, S. N. Blair, *et al.* "Increased Exercise Level and Plasma Lipoprotein Concentrations: A One-Year, Randomized, Controlled Study in Sedentary, Middle-Aged Men." *Metabolism* 32:31–39, 1983.

Wood, P. D., W. Haskell, H. Klein, *et al.* "The Distribution of Plasma Lipoproteins in Middle-Aged Male Runners." *Metabolism* 25:1249–1257, 1976.

Work, J. "Does Physical Fitness Lengthen Life?" *The Physician and Sportsmedicine* 16:15–16, 1988.

Yang, M. U., and T. B. Van Itallie. "Composition of Weight Lost During Short-term Weight Reduction." *Journal of Clinical Investigation* 58:722–730, 1976.

Zukel, W. J., R. H. Lewis, P. E. Enterline, *et al.* "A Short-term Community Study of the Epidemiology of Coronary Heart Disease: A Preliminary Report on the North Dakota Study." *American Journal of Public Health* 49:1630–1639, 1959.

Part II

Aniansson, A., M. Hedberg, G. B. Henning, *et al*. "Muscle Morphology, Enzymatic Activity, and Muscle Strength in Elderly Men: A Follow-up Study." *Muscle Nerve* 9:585–591, 1986.

Aniansson, A., G. Grimby, M. Hedberg, *et al*. "Muscle Morphology, Enzyme Activity and Muscle Strength in Elderly Men and Women." *Clinical Physiology* 1:73–86, 1981.

Aniansson, A., and E. Gustafsson. "Physical Training in Elderly Men with Special Reference to Quadriceps Muscle Strength and Morphology." *Clinical Physiology* 1:87–98, 1981.

Aniansson, A., G. Grimby, and A. Rundgren. "Isometric and Isokinetic Quadriceps Muscle Strength in 70-Year-Old Men and Women." *Scandinavian Journal of Rehabilitative Medicine* 12:161–168, 1980.

Ball, M. F., J. J. Canary, and L. H. Kyle. "Comparative Effects of Caloric Restriction and Total Starvation on Body Composition in Obesity." *Annals Internal Medicine* 67:60–67, 1967.

Ballor, D. L., V. L. Katch, M. D. Becque, *et al*. "Resistance Weight Training During Caloric Restriction Enhances Lean Body Weight Maintenance." *American Journal of Clinical Nutrition* 47:19–25, 1988.

Bar-Or, O., H. M. Lundegren, and E. R. Buskirk. "Heat Tolerance of Exercising Obese and Lean Women." *Journal of Applied Physiology* 26: 403–409, 1969.

Barry, H. C. "Exercise Prescriptions for the Elderly." *American Family Physicians* 34:155–162, 1986.

Blackburn, G. L., and B. S. Kanders. "Medical Evaluation and Treatment of the Obese Patient with Cardiovascular Disease." *American Journal of Cardiology* 60:55G–58G, 1987.

Borkan, G. A., D. E. Hults, A. F. Gerzof, *et al*. "Age Changes in Body Composition Revealed by Computer Tomography." *Journal of Gerontology* 38:673–677, 1983.

Brooks, G. A., and T. D. Fahey. *Exercise Physiology: Human Bioenergetics and Its Applications*. New York: John Wiley & Sons, Inc., 1984.

Brownell, K. D. "Obesity: Understanding and Treating a Serious, Prevalent, and Refactory Disorder." *Journal of Consulting and Clinical Psychology* 50(6):820–840, 1982.

Bureau of Labor Statistics. *Employment and Earnings*. Washington, DC: U.S. Government Printing Office, November, 1986.

Buskirk, E. R., R. H. Thompson, L. Lutwak, *et al*. "Energy Balance of Obese Patients During Weight Reduction: Influence of Diet Restriction and Exercise." *Annals of the New York Academy of Science* 110:918–940, 1963.

Caccia, M. R., J. B. Harris, and M. A. Johnson. "Morphology and Physiology of Skeletal Muscle in Aging Rodents." *Muscle Nerve* 2:202–212, 1979.

Campbell, M. J., A. J. McComas, and F. Petito. "Physiological Changes in Aging Muscles," *Journal of Neurology, Neurosurgery and Psychiatry* 36:174–182, 1973.

Caspersen, C. J., G. M. Christenson, and R. A. Pollard. "Status of the 1990 Physical Fitness and Exercise Objectives—Evidence from NHIS 1985." *Public Health Report* 101:587–592, 1986.

Chapman, E. A., H. A. de Vries, and R. Swezey. "Joint Stiffness: Effects of Exercise on Young and Old Men." *Journal of Gerontology* 27:218–221, 1972.

Daw, C. K., J. W. Starnes, and T. P. White. "Muscle Atrophy and Hypoplasia with Aging: Impact of Training and Food Restriction." *Journal of Applied Physiology* 64:2428–2432, 1988.

Dietz, W. H., Jr., and S. L. Gortmaker. "Do We Fatten Our Children at the Television Set? Obesity and Television Viewing in Children and Adolescents." *Pediatrics* 75:807–812, 1985.

Drinkwater, B. D., K. L. Nilson, and C. S. Chestnut III. "Bone Mineral Content of Amenorrheic and Eumenorrheic Athletes." *New England Journal of Medicine* 311:277–281, 1984.

Durrant, M. L., J. S. Garrow, P. Royston, *et al*. "Factors Influencing the Composition of the Weight Lost by Obese Patients on a Reducing Diet." *British Journal of Nutrition* 44:275–285, 1980.

Garn, S. M. "Bone Loss and Aging." In R. Goldman and M. Rockstein (eds.), *The Physiology and Pathology of Aging*. New York: Academic Press, pp. 281–299, 1975.

Garrow, J. S. "Effect of Exercise on Obesity." *Acta Medica Scandinavica* Suppl. 711:67–73, 1986.

Greenleaf, J. E. "Physiological Responses to Prolonged Bed Rest and Fluid Immersion in Humans." *Journal of Applied Physiology* 57:619–633, 1984.

Grimby, G. "Physical Activity and Effects of Muscle Training in the Elderly." *Annals of Clinical Research* 20:62–66, 1988.

Grimby, G., and B. Saltin. "Mini-Review. The Aging Muscle." *Clinical Physiology*. 3:209–218, 1983.

Grimby, G., B. Danneskiold-Samsoe, K. Hvid, *et al*. "Morphology and

Enzymatic Capacity in Arm and Leg Muscles in 78–81-Year-Old Men and Women." *Acta Physiologica Scandinavica* 115:125–34, 1982.

Groves, D. "Is Childhood Obesity Related to TV Addiction?" *The Physician and Sportsmedicine* 16:117–122, 1988.

Hooper, A. C. B. "Length, Diameter and Number of Aging Skeletal Muscle Fibres." *Gerontology* 27:121–126, 1981.

Katch, V., M. D. Becque, C. Marks, *et al.* "Oxygen Uptake and Energy Output During Walking of Obese Male and Female Adolescents." *American Journal of Clinical Nutrition* 47:26–32, 1988.

Kukkonen-Harjula, K. "More Exercise for the Obese?" *Annals of Clinical Research* 20:67–70, 1988.

Kuntzleman, C. T. *Activetics*, New York: Peter Wyden, Publisher, 1975.

Larsson, L. "Histochemical Characteristics of Human Skeletal Muscle During Aging." *Acta Physiologica Scandinavica* 117:469–471, 1983.

Larsson, L., B. Sjodin, and J. Karlsson. "Histochemical and Biochemical Changes in Human Skeletal Muscle with Age in Sedentary Males, Age 22–65 Years." *Acta Physiologica Scandinavica* 103:31–39, 1978.

Larsson, L., and J. Karlsson. "Isometric and Dynamic Endurance as a Function of Age and Skeletal Muscle Characteristics." *Acta Physiologica Scandinavica* 104:129–136, 1978.

Lexell, J., K. Henriksson-Larsson, B. Wimblad, *et al.* "Distribution of Different Fiber Types in Human Skeletal Muscle. 3. Effects of Aging in M. Vastus Lateralis Studies in Whole Muscle Cross-Sections." *Muscle Nerve* 6:588–595, 1983.

McArdle, W. D., F. I. Katch, V. L. Katch. *Exercise Physiology: Energy, Nutrition, and Human Performance*, 2nd edition. Philadelphia: Lea & Febiger, Publisher, 1986.

McCarter, R. J. M., and J. McGee. "Influence of Nutrition and Aging on the Composition and Function of Rat Skeletal Muscle." *Journal of Gerontology* 42:432–441, 1987.

McCarter, R. J. M., E. J. Masoro, and B. P. Yu. "Rat Muscle Structure and Metabolism in Relation to Age and Food Intake." *American Journal of Physiology* 242:R89–R93, 1982.

Mayhew, J. L., and P. M. Gross. "Body Composition Changes in Young Women with High Resistence Weight Training." *Research Quarterly* 45:433–440, 1974.

Miller, J. F., and B. A. Stamford. "Energy Cost of Weighted Walking Versus Jogging for Men and Women." *Journal Applied Physiology* 62:1497–1501, 1987.

Montoye, H. J., and D. E. Lamphiear. "Grip and Arm Strength in Males and Females, Age 10 to 69." *Research Quarterly* 48:109–120, 1977.

Munns, K. "Effects of Exercise on the Range of Joint Motion in Elderly Subjects." In E. L. Smith and R. C. Serfass (eds.), *Exercise and Aging: The Scientific Basis.* Hillside, NJ: Enslow Publishers, 1981, pp. 167–178.

"1988 Report on Television." Northbrook, IL.: Nielsen Media Research, 1988, pp. 8–9.

Passmore, R., and J. V. G. A. Durnin. "Human Energy Expenditure." *Physiological Reviews* 35:801–840, 1955.

Patrick, J. M., E. J. Bassey, and P. H. Fentem. "Changes in Body Fat and Muscle in Manual Workers at and After Retirement." *European Journal of Applied Physiology* 49:187–196, 1982.

Pavlou, K. N., W. P. Steffee, R. H. Lerman, *et al.* "Effects of Dieting and Exercise on Lean Body Mass, Oxygen Uptake, and Strength." *Medical Science in Sports and Exercise* 17:466–71, 1985.

Phinney, S. D., B. M. LaGrange, M. O'Connell, *et al.* "Effects of Aerobic Exercise on Energy Expenditure and Nitrogen Balance During Very Low Calorie Dieting." *Metabolism* 37(8):758–765, 1988.

Sheldahl, L. "Special Ergometric Techniques and Weight Reduction." *Medicine and Science in Sports and Exercise* 18(1):25–30, 1986.

Shock, N. W. "Physiological Aspects of Aging in Man." *Annual Reviews of Physiology* 23:97–122, 1961.

Shock, N. W., D. M. Watkin, M. J. Yiengst, *et al.* "Age Differences in the Water Content of the Body as Related to Basal Oxygen Consumption in Males." *Journal of Gerontology* 18:1–8, 1963.

Sikand, G., A. Kondo, J. P. Foreyt, *et al.* "Two-Year Follow-up of Patients Treated with a Very-Low-Calorie Diet and Exercise Training." *Journal of American Dietetic Association* 88(4):487–488, 1988.

Smith, E. L., W. Reddan, and P. E. Smith. "Physical Activity and Calcium Modalities for Bone Mineral Increase in Aged Women." *Medical Science and Sports Exercise* 13:60–64, 1981.

Smith, E. L., and W. Reddan. "Physical Activity—a Modality for Bone Accretion in the Aged." *American Journal of Roentgenology* 126:1297, 1977. (abstract)

Smith, E. L. "Exercise for Prevention of Osteoporosis: A Review." *The Physician and Sportsmedicine* 10:72–83, 1982.

Smith, E. L., and C. Gilligan. "Physical Activity for the Older Adult." *The Physician and Sportsmedicine* 11:91–101, 1983.

Stamford, B. A. "Exercise and the Elderly." In K. B. Pandolf (ed.), *Exercise and Sports Sciences Reviews*. New York: Macmillan Publishing Co., 16:341–379, 1988.

Stamford, B. A. "Effects of Chronic Institutionalization on the Physical Working Capacity and Trainability of Geriatric Men." *Journal of Gerontology* 28:441–446, 1973.

Stamford, B. A. "Physiological Effects of Training upon Institutionalized Geriatric Men." *Journal of Gerontology* 27:451–455, 1972.

Suominen, H., E. Heikkinen, P. Vainio, *et al.* "Mineral Density of Calcaneus in Men at Different Ages: A Population Study with Special Reference to Life-Style Factors." *Age and Aging* 13:273–281, 1984.

Tremblay, A., J. P. Despres, and C. Bouchard. "The Effects of Exercise Training on Energy Balance and Adipose Tissue Morphology." *Sports Medicine* 2:223–233, 1985.

Wilmore, J. H. "Alterations in Strength, Body Composition, and Anthropometric Measurements Consequent to a 10-Week Weight Training Program." *Medicine and Science in Sports* 6:133–138, 1974.

Young, C. M., S. S. Scanlan, H. S. Im, *et al.* "Effect on Body Composition and Other Parameters in Obese Young Men of Carbohydrate Level of Reduction Diet." *American Journal of Clinical Nutrition* 24:290–296, 1971.

Part III

Abraham, S., C. L. Johnson, and M. F. Najjar. "Weight by Height and Age for Adults 18–74 Years. United States 1971–74." Hyattsville, MD: National Center for Health Statistics, 1979. (*Vital and Health Statistics*, series 11: Data from the National Health Survey #208 [DHEW publication # (PHS) 79-1656.])

Acheson, K. J., Y. Schutz, T. Bessard, *et al.* "Nutritional Influences on Lipogenesis and Thermogenesis After a Carbohydrate Meal." *American Journal of Physiology* 246(9):E62–E70, 1984.

Acheson, K. J., J. P. Flatt, and E. Jequier. "Glycogen Synthesis Versus Lipogenesis After a 500-Gram Carbohydrate Meal in Man." *Metabolism* 31:1234–1240, 1982.

Adams, C. E., and K. J. Morgan. "Periodicity of Eating: Implications for Human Food Consumption." *Nutrition Research* 1:525–550, 1981.

Anderson, J. W. *Plant Fiber in Foods*. Lexington, KY: HCF Diabetes Research Foundation, Inc., 1986.

Anholm, A. C. "The Relationship of a Vegetarian Diet and Blood Pressure." *Preventive Medicine* 4:35, 1975.

Armstrong, B., A. J. Van Merwyk, and H. Coates. "Blood Pressure in Seventh-

Day Adventist Vegetarians." *American Journal of Epidemiology* 105:444–449, 1977.

Arner, P., P. Engfeldt, and H. Lithell. "Site Differences in the Basal Metabolism of Subcutaneous Fat in Obese Women." *Journal of Clinical Endocrinology Metabolism* 53:948–952, 1981.

Berry, E. M., J. Hirsch, J. Most, *et al*. "The Role of Dietary Fat in Human Obesity." *International Journal of Obesity* 10:123–31, 1986.

Bjorntorp, P. "Hazards in Subgroups of Human Obesity." *European Journal of Clinical Investigation* 14:239–241, 1984.

Blair, D., J. P. Habicht, E. A. H. Sims, *et al*. "Evidence for an Increased Risk for Hypertension with Centrally Located Body Fat and the Effect of Race and Sex on This Risk." *American Journal of Epidemiology* 119:526–540, 1984.

Bray, G. A., B. J. Whipp, and S. N. Koyal. "The Acute Effects of Food Intake on Energy Expenditure During Cycle Ergometry." *American Journal of Clinical Nutrition* 27:254–259, 1974.

Bray, G. A. "Lipogenesis in Human Adipose Tissue: Some Effects of Nibbling and Gorging." *Journal of Clinical Investigation* 51:537–548, 1972.

Broeder, C. E., M. Branner, Z. Hofman, *et al*. "The Metabolic Consequences of Low and Moderate Intensity Exercise with or Without Feeding in Lean Males." *Medicine and Science in Sports and Exercise* 20(2 Suppl.):150, 1988. (Abstract)

Brody, J. *Jane Brody's Nutrition Book*. New York: W. W. Norton & Company Publishers, 1981.

Cahill, G. F., Jr., M. G. Herrera, A. P. Morgan, *et al*. "Hormone-Fuel Interrelationships During Fasting." *Journal of Clinical Investigation* 45:1751–1769, 1966.

Carlsson, L. A., J. Boberg, and B. Hogstedt. "Some Physiological and Clinical Implications of Lipid Mobilization from Adipose Tissue." *Handbook of Physiology* (Sect. 5):625–644, 1965.

Crapo, P. A., G. M. Reaven, and J. M. Olefsky. "Plasma Glucose and Insulin Responses to Orally Administered Simple and Complex Carbohydrates." *Diabetes* 25:741–747, 1976.

Despres, J. P., A. Tremblay, A. Nadeau, *et al*. "Physical Training and Changes in Regional Adipose Tissue Distribution." *Acta Medica Scandinavica*, Suppl. 723:205–212, 1988.

Despres, J. P., C. Allard, A. Tremblay, *et al*. "Evidence for a Regional Component of Body Fatness in the Association with Serum Lipids in Men and Women." *Metabolism* 34(10):967–973, 1985.

Dreon, D. M., B. Frey-Hewitt, N. Ellsworth, *et al*. "Dietary Fat: Carbohydrate Ratio and Obesity in Middle-Aged Men." *American Journal of Clinical Nutrition* 47:995–1000, 1988.

Drewnowski, A., J. D. Brunzell, K. Sande, *et al.* "Sweet Tooth Reconsidered: Taste Responsiveness in Human Obesity." *Physiology and Behavior* 35:617–622, 1985.

Duncan, K. H., J. A. Bacon, and R. L. Weinsier. "The Effects of High and Low Energy Density Diets on Satiety, Energy Intake, and Eating Time of Obese and Non-Obese Subjects." *American Journal of Clinical Nutrition* 37:763–767, 1983.

Eichner, E. R. "Antithrombotic Effects of Exercise." *American Family Physician* 36(5):207–211, 1987.

Evans, D. J., R. G. Hoffmann, R. K. Kalkhoff, *et al.* "Relationship of Body Fat Topography to Insulin Sensitivity and Metabolic Profiles in Premenopausal Women." *Metabolism* 33:68–75, 1984.

Fabry, P., J. Fodor, A. Hejl, *et al.* "The Frequency of Meals: Its Relation to Overweight, Hypercholesterolemia, and Decreased Glucose-Tolerance. *Lancet* 2:614–615, 1964.

Fabry, P., E. Horakova, E. Konopasek, *et al.* "Energy Metabolism and Growth in Rats Adapted to Intermittent Starvation." *British Journal of Nutrition* 17:295–301, 1963.

Fixx, J. *The Complete Book of Running.* New York: Random House, 1977.

Flatt, J. P. "Dietary Fat, Carbohydrate Balance, and Weight Maintenance: Effects of Exercise." *American Journal of Clinical Nutrition* 45:296–306, 1987.

Flatt, J. P., E. Ravussin, K. J. Acheson, *et al.* "Effects of Dietary Fat on Postprandial Substrate Oxidation and on Carbohydrate and Fat Balances." *Journal of Clinical Investigation* 76:1019–1024, 1985.

Friedman, M. I., and I. Ramirez. "Insulin Counteracts the Satiating Effect of a Fat Meal in Rats." *Physiology and Behavior* (40):655–659, 1987.

Friedman, M. I., and I. Ramirez. "Relationship of Fat Metabolism to Food Intake." *American Journal of Clinical Nutrition* 42:1093–1098, 1985.

Galli, C. "Dietary Influences on Prostaglandin Synthesis." *Advances in Nutrition Research* 3:95–126, 1980.

Goodnight, S. H., Jr., W. S. Harris, W. E. Connor, *et al.* "Polyunsaturated Fatty Acids, Hyperlipidemia, and Thrombosis." *Arteriosclerosis* 2:87–113, 1982.

Golay, A., J. P. Felber, H. U. Meyer, *et al.* "Study on Lipid Metabolism in Obesity Diabetes." *Metabolism* 33:111–116, 1984.

Goldberg, A. P., and P. J. Coon. "Non-Insulin-Dependent Diabetes Mellitus in the Elderly: Influence of Obesity and Physical Inactivity." *Endocrinology and Metabolism Clinics* 16(4):843–865, 1987.

Grey, N., and D. M. Kipnis. "Effect of Diet Composition on the Hyperinsulinemia of Obesity." *New England Journal of Medicine* 285:827–831, 1971.

Harsha Rao, R., U. Brahmaji Rao, and S. G. Srikantia. "Effect of Polyunsaturated Rich Vegetable Oils on Blood Pressure in Essential Hypertension." *Clinical Experimental Hypertension* 3:27–38, 1981.

Hartz, A. J., D. C. Rupley, Jr., R. D. Kalkhoff, *et al.* "Relationship of Obesity to Diabetes: Influence of Obesity Level and Body Fat Distribution." *Preventive Medicine* 12:351–357, 1983.

Heaton, K. W. "Food Fiber as an Obstacle to Energy Intake." *Lancet* 2:1418–21, 1973.

Heaton, K. W., S. N. Marcus, P. M. Emmett, *et al.* "Particle Size of Wheat, Maize, and Oat Test Meals: Effects on Plasma Glucose and Insulin Responses and on the Rate of Starch Digestion in Vitro." *American Journal of Clinical Nutrition* 47:675–682, 1988.

Iacono, J. M., M. W. Marshall, R. M. Dougherty, *et al.* "Reduction in Blood Pressure Associated with High Polyunsaturated Fat Diets That Reduce Blood Cholesterol in Man." *Preventive Medicine* 4:426–433, 1975.

Jacobson, B. K., K. Trygg, I. Hjermann, *et al.* "Acyl Pattern of Adipose Tissue Triglycerides, Plasma Free Fatty Acids, and Diet of a Group of Men Participating in a Primary Coronary Prevention Program (the Oslo Study)." *American Journal of Clinical Nutrition* 38:906–913, 1983.

Jiang, C. L., and J. N. Hunt. "The Relation Between Freely Chosen Meals and Body Habitus." *American Journal of Clinical Nutrition* 38:32–40, 1983.

Kalkhoff, R. K., A. H. Hartz, D. Rupley, *et al.* "Relationship of Body Fat Distribution to Blood Pressure, Carbohydrate Tolerance, and Plasma Lipids in Healthy Obese Women." *J. Lab. Clin. Med.* 102(4):621–627, 1983.

Kanarek, R. B., and E. Hirsch. "Dietary-Induced Overeating in Experimental Animals." *Federation Proceedings* 36(2):154–158, 1977.

Katahn, M. *The T-Factor Diet.* New York: W. W. Norton, 1989.

Katch, F. I., P. M. Clarkson, W. Kroll, *et al.* "Effects of Sit Up Exercise Training on Adipose Cell Size and Adiposity." *Research Quarterly for Exercise and Sport* 55:242–247, 1984.

Keeling, W. F., and B. J. Martin. "Gastrointestinal Transit During Mild Exercise." *Journal of Applied Physiology* 63(3):978–981, 1987.

Kissebah, A. H., N. Vydelingum, R. Murray, *et al.* "Relation of Body Fat Distribution to Metabolic Complications of Obesity." *Journal of Clinical Endocrinology and Metabolism* 54(1):254–260, 1982.

Kraegen, E. W., D. E. James, L. H. Storlien, *et al.* "In Vivo Insulin Resistance in Individual Peripheral Tissues of the High-Fat-Fed Rat: Assessment by Euglycemic Clamp Plus Deoxyglucose Administration." *Diabetologia* 29:192–197, 1986.

Kreisberg, R. A., B. R. Boshell, and J. DiPlacido, et al. "Insulin Secretion in Obesity." *New England Journal of Medicine* 276:314–319, 1967.

Krotkiewski, M., P. Bjorntrop, L. Sjostrom, et al. "Impact of Obesity on Metabolism in Men and Women: Importance of Regional Adipose Tissue Distribution." *Journal of Clinical Investigation* 72:1150–1162, 1983.

Leon, A. S. "Physiological Interactions Between Diet and Exercise in the Etiology and Prevention of Ischaemic Heart Disease." *Annals of Clinical Research* 20:114–120, 1988.

Leveille, G. A. "Adipose Tissue Metabolism: Influence of Periodicity of Eating and Diet Composition." *Federation Proceedings* 29:1294–1301, 1970.

Lissner, L., D. A. Levitsky, B. J. Strupp, et al. "Dietary Fat and the Regulation of Energy Intake in Human Subjects." *American Journal of Clinical Nutrition* 46:886–892, 1987.

Men's Health Newsletter. "Another Slap in the Face for Saturated Fat." January 1989, p. 3.

Men's Health Newsletter. "Oat Bran Cheaper Than Drugs for Cutting Cholesterol." September 1988, p. 1.

Men's Health Newsletter. "Green Light for Splurging." September 1988, p. 8.

Metzner, H. L., D. D. Lamphiear, N. C. Wheeler, et al. "The Relationship Between Frequency of Eating and Adiposity in Adult Men and Women in the Tecumseh Community Health Study." *American Journal of Clinical Nutrition* 30:712–715, 1979.

Miller, D. S., and P. Mumford, "Gluttony, I. An Experimental Study of Overeating Low- and High-Protein Diets." *American Journal of Clinical Nutrition* 20:1212–1222, 1967.

Miller, D. S., P. Mumford, and M. J. Stock. "Gluttony 2. Thermogenesis in Overeating Man." *American Journal of Clinical Nutrition* 20:1223–1229, 1967.

National Institutes of Health Consensus Development. *Diet and Exercise in Noninsulin-Dependent Diabetes Mellitus.* Vol. 6, No. 8. December 10, 1986.

Oscai, L. B., W. C. Miller, and D. A. Arnall. "Effects of Dietary Sugar and of Dietary Fat on Food Intake and Body Fat Content in Rats." *Growth* 51:64–73, 1987.

Oscai, L. B., and W. C. Miller. "Dietary-Induced Severe Obesity: Exercise Implications." *Medicine and Science in Sports and Exercise* 18(1):6–9, 1985.

Oscai, L. B., M. M. Brown, and W. C. Miller. "Effect of Dietary Fat on Food Intake, Growth and Body Composition in Rats." *Growth* 48:415–424, 1984.

Oscai, L. B. "Dietary-Induced Severe Obesity: A Rat Model." *American Journal of Physiology* 242:R212–R215, 1982.

Paoletti, R., C. Galli, E. Agradi, *et al.* "Influence of Dietary Essential Fatty Acids (EFA) on the Prostaglandin System and Its Role in Platelet Function." In: Aebi, Brubacher, Turner (eds.), *Problems in Nutrition Research Today.* London: Academic Press, Inc., 1981, 93–100.

Porikos, K. P., M. F. Hesser, and T. B. Van Itallie. "Caloric Regulation in Normal-Weight Men Maintained on a Palatable Diet of Conventional Foods." *Physiology and Behavior* 28:293–300, 1982.

Porikos, K. P., G. Booth, and T. B. Van Itallie. "Effects of Covert Nutritive Dilution on the Spontaneous Food Intake of Obese Individuals: A Pilot Study." *American Journal of Clinical Nutrition* 30:1638–1644, 1977.

Puka, P., A. Nissinen, E. Vartiainen, *et al.* "Controlled Randomized Trial of the Effect of Dietary Fat on Blood Pressure." *Lancet* I:1–10, 1983.

Rogers, P. J., and J. E. Blundell. "Meal Patterns and Food Selection During the Development of Obesity in Rats Fed a Cafeteria Diet." *Neuroscience Behavior Review* 8:441–453, 1984.

Romieu, I., W. C. Willett, M. J. Stampfer, *et al.* "Energy Intake and Other Determinants of Relative Weight." *American Journal of Clinical Nutrition* 46:406–412, 1988.

Rothwell, N. J., and M. J. Stock. "Regulation of Energy Balance." *Annual Review of Nutrition* 1:235–256, 1981.

Rouse, I. L., L. J. Beilin, B. K. Armstrong, *et al.* "Blood-Pressure-Lowering Effect of a Vegetarian Diet: Controlled Trial in Normotensive Subjects." *Lancet* 5–10, January 1/8, 1983.

Sacks, F. M., B. Rosner, and E. H. Kass. "Blood Pressure in Vegetarians." *American Journal of Epidemiology* 100:390–398, 1974.

Sadur, C. N., T. J. Yost, and R. H. Eckel. "Fat Feeding Decreases Insulin Responsiveness of Adipose Tissue Lipoprotein Lipase." *Metabolism* 33:1043–1047, 1984.

Salmon, D. M., and J. P. Flatt. "Effect of Dietary Fat Content on the Incidence of Obesity Among ad Libitum Fed Mice." *International Journal of Obesity* 9:443–449, 1985.

Schemmel R., O. Mickelsen, and K. Motawi. "Conversion of Dietary Body Energy in Rats as Affected by Strain, Sex and Ration." *Journal of Nutrition* 102:1187–97, 1972.

Schlierf, G., and H. Raetzer. "Diurnal Patterns of Blood Sugar, Plasma Insulin, Free Fatty Acids and Triglyceride Levels in Normal Subjects and in Patients with Type IV Hyperlipoproteinemia, and the Effect of Meal Frequency." *Nutrition and Metabolism* 14:113–126, 1972.

Segal, K. R., E. Presta, and B. Gutin. "Thermic Effect of Food During Graded Exercise in Normal Weight and Obese Men." *American Journal of Clinical Nutrition* 40:995–1000, 1984.

Select Committee on Nutrition and Human Needs, U.S. Senate. *Dietary Goals for the United States,* 2nd ed. Washington, DC: U.S. Government Printing Office, 1977. (U.S. Department of Agriculture Handbook #504).

Senate Select Committee on Nutrition and Human Needs. *Dietary Goals for the US—Supplemental Views.* Washington, DC: U.S. Government Printing Office, 1977.

Sims, E. A. H., and E. Danforth. "Expenditure and Storage of Energy in Man." *Journal of Clinical Investigation* 79:1019–1025, 1987.

Smith, T. K., R. M. Otto, J. W. Wygand, *et al.* "The Effect of Exercise and Food Ingestion upon Basal Metabolism." *Medicine and Science in Sports and Exercise* 18(2)450, 1986. (Abstract)

Stamford, B. A., S. Matter, R. D. Fell, *et al.* "Effects of Smoking Cessation on Weight Gain, Metabolic Rate, Caloric Consumption and Blood Lipids." *American Journal of Clinical Nutrition* 43:486–494, 1986.

Stern, B., S. Heyden, D. Miller, *et al.* "Intervention Study in High School Students with Elevated Blood Pressures. Dietary Experiment with Polyunsaturated Fatty Acids." *Nutrition Metabolism* 24:137–147, 1980.

Storlien, L. H., D. E. James, K. M. Burleigh, *et al.* "Fat Feeding Causes Widespread in Vivo Insulin Resistance, Decreased Energy Expenditure, and Obesity in Rats." *American Journal Physiology* 251(14): #576–#583, 1986.

Torbay N., E. F. Bracco, A. Geliebter, *et al.* "Insulin Increases Body Fat Despite Control of Food Intake and Physical Activity." *American Journal of Physiology* 248:R120–R124, 1985.

USDA Science and Education Administration. *Nationwide Food Consumption Survey, 1977–78.* Washington, DC: U.S. Government Printing Office, 1980. (Preliminary report #2)

USDA Economics, Statistical and Cooperative Service. *Food Consumption, Prices and Expenditures.* Washington, DC: U.S. Government Printing Office, 1976.

USDA Agriculture Handbook 8-1. *Composition of Foods: Dairy and Egg Products—Raw, Processed, Prepared.* November 1976.

USDA Agriculture Handbook 8-4. *Composition of Foods: Fats and Oils—Raw, Processed, Prepared.* Science and Education Administration. June 1979.

USDA Agriculture Handbook 8-5. *Composition of Foods: Poultry Products—Raw, Processed, Prepared.* Human Nutrition Information. August 1979.

USDA Agriculture Handbook 8-6. *Composition of Foods: Soups, Sauces, and Gravies—Raw, Processed, Prepared.* Science and Education Administration. February 1980.

USDA Agriculture Handbook 8-8. *Composition of Foods: Breakfast Cereals—Raw, Processed, Prepared.* Human Nutrition Information. July 1982.

USDA Agriculture Handbook 8-9. *Composition of Foods: Fruit and Fruit Juices —Raw, Processed, Prepared.* Human Nutrition Information. August 1982.

USDA Agriculture Handbook 8-10. *Composition of Foods: Pork Products— Raw, Processed, Prepared.* Human Nutrition Information. August 1983.

USDA Agriculture Handbook 8-11. *Composition of Foods: Vegetable and Vegetable Products—Raw, Processed, Prepared.* Human Nutrition Information. August 1984.

USDA Agriculture Handbook 8-12. *Composition of Foods: Nut and Seed Products—Raw, Processed, Prepared.* Human Nutrition Information. September 1984.

USDA Agriculture Handbook 8-13. *Composition of Foods: Beef Products—Raw, Processed, Prepared.* Human Nutrition Information. August 1986.

USDA Agriculture Handbook 8-15. *Composition of Foods: Finfish and Shellfish Products—Raw, Processed, Prepared.* September 1987.

USDA Agriculture Handbook 8-16. *Composition of Foods: Legumes and Legume Products—Raw, Processed, Prepared.* Human Nutrition Information. December 1986.

USDA Agriculture Handbook 8-21. *Composition of Foods: Fast Foods.* Human Nutrition Information. September 1988.

USDA Agriculture Handbook 456. *Nutritive Value of American Foods.* November 1975.

USDA Home and Garden Bulletin. *Nutritive Value of Foods.* No. 72. Human Nutrition Information Service, 1986.

U.S. Dept. of Health and Human Services. *Eating to Lower Your High Blood Cholesterol.* NIH Publication No. 87–2920, September 1987.

Vague, J. "The Degree of Masculine Differentiation of Obesities, a Factor Determining Predisposition to Diabetes, Atherosclerosis, Gout and Uric Calculous Disease." *American Journal of Clinical Nutrition* 4:20–34, 1956.

Van Itallie, T. B. "Dietary Fiber and Obesity." *American Journal of Clinical Nutrition* 31:543–52, 1978.

Whitney, E. N., C. B. Cataldo, and S. R. Rolfes. *Understanding Normal and Clinical Nutrition,* 2nd edition. New York: West Publishing Co., 1987.

Part IV

Benson, H. *The Relaxation Response.* New York: Avon Books, 1975.

Harris, T. G. "Heart Disease in Retreat." *Psychology Today* 23:46–48, 1989.

Lakein, A. *How to Get Control of Your Life and Time.* New York: New American Library, 1973.

Pearsall, P. *Super Immunity: Master Your Emotions and Improve Your Health.* New York: Fawcett Gold Medal, 1987.

Vaillant, G. E. "Natural History of Male Psychologic Health: Effects of Mental Health on Physical Health." *New England Journal of Medicine* 301:1249–1254, 1979.

Williams, R. *The Trusting Heart: Great News About Type A Behavior.* New York: Random House, 1989.

APPENDIX

Fitness in the Kitchen: Lipo-Fit Recipes

Stamford

Joy, my wife, agreed to write down many of the recipes that deserve much of the credit for rescuing me from my errant eating habits of old. They are delicious, yet low in fat (saturated fat especially), low in calories, low in cholesterol, low in sodium, and low in refined sugar.

As a busy professional who views cooking as a necessity, not an art, Joy prefers dishes that are quick and easy, as well as exceptionally nutritious. None here requires more than about twenty minutes of actual preparation, and there is very little cleanup, thanks to their low fat (grease) content. All recipes have been analyzed using the *Auto-Nutritionist III* computer program produced by N-Squared Computing, of Silverton, Oregon.

☐ *A word on seasonings*: Feel free to experiment and alter seasonings according to personal preferences. As you'll see, Joy and I are partial to the Mediterranean flavors of garlic and basil, but let your own tastes be your guide.

Note, too, that in a few cases—the cabbage salad, for example—total calories are so low that the use of even a single teaspoon of oil yields a high fat percentage. You're still getting a very low *amount* of fat in this recipe, however, as indicated by the actual grams of fat per serving, so don't be concerned.

Breads and Muffins*

Easy Non-Yeasted Whole Wheat Bread

3½ cups whole-wheat flour
1–2 tsp. all-phosphate baking powder
1 tsp. salt
1 cup whole-wheat berries, cooked (optional)
1½ –2 cups skim milk
1 tsp. honey or 1 Tbsp. blackstrap molasses (optional)
1 egg + 1 Tbsp. water

Mix dry ingredients. Add wheat berries and stir. Add honey or molasses to milk. Add milk to flour mixture—just enough to make a moist dough. Knead a few times. Make a round or oblong loaf, slice a large **X** through center top. Beat egg with fork and add water; brush on loaf. (You will use very little of the egg-water mixture.) Place on lightly greased sheet and bake in preheated 450-degree oven for 15 minutes; turn heat down to 350 degrees and bake for another 20–30 minutes or until done.

Makes a great "chewy" loaf of bread and it's very filling. It will rise a little more with molasses or honey than without.

Total working time: 5–8 minutes

20 slices = 40 half-slice servings			
½ slice = 41.6 calories (without honey or berries)			
Protein 18%; carbohydrate 75%; fat 7%.			
Sat. fat	.10 gm.	Cholesterol	7.1 mg.
Mono. fat	.06 gm.	Fiber	1.3 gm.
Poly. fat	.02 gm.	Sodium	68.09 mg.

---

*Note that all breads and muffins call for *all-phosphate baking powder*. Most baking powders contain sodium and aluminum. All-phosphate powders contain neither and are available in natural food stores and some supermarkets. I use *Rumford* brand.

Variations:
1. Substitute 1 tsp. baking soda for baking powder, skim buttermilk for skim milk, add ½ cup raisins instead of wheat berries, and you have a whole wheat Irish Soda Bread.
2. Add 1 cup oat bran or oat flour and a little more milk. The oats keep the bread moist. (See next recipe.)
3. To increase protein value, add 1 cup soy flour or soy grits and more milk. (Soy complements wheat to make a complete protein.)

—

Whole Wheat/Oat Bran Bread

—

3½ cups stone-ground whole-wheat bread flour
1 cup oat bran
2 tsp. all-phosphate baking powder
1 tsp. salt
1 Tbsp. Brewer's yeast and/or wheat germ
1 cup wheat berries, cooked
1 Tbsp. blackstrap molasses
2¼ cups skim milk (or more, as needed)
1 egg and 1 Tbsp. water

Proceed as in preceding recipe.

20 slices = 40 half-slice servings	
½ slice = 56 calories per half slice.	
Protein 18%; carbohydrate 74%; fat 8%.	
Sat. fat .06 gm.	Cholesterol .28 mg.
Mono. fat .01 gm.	Fiber 1.705 gm.
Poly. fat .00 gm.	Sodium 94.18 mg.

You'll notice that the following muffin recipes have less oil than usual muffin recipes and no sugar. We think they are delicious, but they are not the usual sweet and oil-rich muffins. Eat them with a little apple butter or all-fruit preserves instead of butter or margarine.

No-Oil Oat Bran Muffins

2 cups oat bran
½ cup whole-wheat flour
2 tsp. all-phosphate baking powder
¼ –1 tsp. salt (optional)
1¾ cup skim milk
2 egg whites

Mix dry ingredients. Mix milk and egg whites. Blend into dry
ingredients. Spoon into lightly greased 12-pocket muffin tin. (Use no
more than ½ tsp. corn or safflower oil margarine for all 12 cups, or use
a non-aerosol cooking spray.) Bake at 400–425 degrees for 20–25
minutes or until lightly browned.

Makes 12 muffins at 88 calories each Protein 24%; carbohydrate 62%; fat 14%		
Sat. fat .08 gm.	Cholesterol	13.7 mg.
Mono. fat .02 gm.	Fiber	3.1 gm.
Poly. fat .01 gm.	Sodium	180.9 mg.

Variations:
1. Add 4 tsp. cinnamon, ⅛ tsp. ginger, ¼ tsp. clove, and ¼ tsp.
   nutmeg to dry ingredients for cinnamon-spice muffins.
2. Add 4 Tbsp. nonfat dry milk powder, to increase protein values.
3. Add 1 Tbsp. blackstrap molasses and/or brewer's yeast or wheat germ
   to increase nutrients. *Note:* Do not confuse regular molasses for
   blackstrap or active yeast for brewer's (nutritional) yeast.
4. Add chopped apples, raisins, or other fruit or seeds.
5. Substitute fruit juices for all or part of the milk.

Oat Flour Muffins

2 cups oat flour*
1 cup whole-wheat flour
2 tsp. all-phosphate baking powder
½ tsp. salt (optional)
2 cups skim milk

See directions for the preceding recipe.

> Makes 16 muffins at 76 calories each.
> Protein 19%; carbohydrate 71%; fat 10%
>
> Sat. fat   .19 gm.   Cholesterol .625 mg.
> Mono. fat .25 gm.   Fiber   1.53 gm.
> Poly. fat   .26 gm.   Sodium   70.44 mg.

Whole Wheat Muffins with Oat Bran

2 cups stone-ground whole-wheat flour
1 cup oatmeal or oat bran
2 tsp. all-phosphate baking powder
½ tsp. salt (optional)
2 tsp. safflower oil (optional)
2 cups skim milk

Grease muffin tin (for 12) with ½ tsp. margarine or non-aerosol cooking spray.

Mix dry ingredients. Mix oil and milk and add, stirring until all is moistened. Add a little more milk if necessary. Spoon into tin, and bake at 425 degrees for 20–25 minutes until a light brown.

Working time: 6–8 minutes

> Makes 12 muffins at 115 calories each
> Protein 18%; carbohydrate 70%; fat 12%
>
> Sat. fat   .28 gm.   Cholesterol .83 mg.
> Mono. fat .27 gm.   Fiber   2.92 gm.
> Poly. fat   .74 gm.   Sodium   175.4 mg.

---

*Oat flour can be made in your blender or processor from oatmeal or oat bran or purchased from a natural food store.

Variations:
1. Use part barley flour, rice flour, etc. or substitute barley or whole-wheat pastry flour for the whole wheat.
2. Add ½ cup nonfat dry milk powder and/or ½ cup soy flour, if you want to enhance protein value.
3. Salt can be omitted if you are on a salt-free diet. Omit oil if you're trying to lose weight. (Oil makes crust tender, but these are very good with no oil. Just be certain not to overbake, as crust will get thicker.)

Simple Wheat and Oat Muffins

2 cups whole-wheat flour
1 cup oat bran, oatmeal, or oat flour
2 tsp. all-phosphate baking powder
½ tsp. salt (optional)
2 cups skim milk

Mix dry ingredients. Add skim milk. Spoon into lightly greased muffin tins. Bake 400–425 degrees for 15–18 minutes.

For variations, see suggestions with preceding recipes.

Makes 16 large muffins at 81 calories each			
Protein 19%; carbohydrate 75%; fat 7%			
Sat. fat	.16 gm.	Cholesterol	.63 mg.
Mono. fat	.13 gm.	Fiber	2.18 gm.
Poly. fat	.13 gm.	Sodium	131.5 mg.

Corn and Wheat Muffins (or Cornbread)

1 cup whole-wheat flour
1 cup stone-ground corn meal
1 tsp. all-phosphate baking powder

½ tsp. salt (optional)
2 tsp. safflower oil
1¼ cups skim milk

Mix dry ingredients. Add oil and milk, adding more milk if necessary. Spoon into lightly greased muffin tin (or round cake pan). Bake at 425 degrees for about 25 minutes or until lightly browned.

> Makes 12 muffins/servings at 87 calories
>   each
> Protein 14%; carbohydrate 72%; fat 14%
>
> | Sat. fat | .19 gm. | Cholesterol | .521 mg. |
> |---|---|---|---|
> | Mono. fat | .11 gm. | Fiber | 1.267 gm. |
> | Poly. fat | .57 gm. | Sodium | 49.63 mg. |

Variation: Make an all-corn muffin by substituting another cup of corn for the wheat. Add 2 egg whites if desired.

Barley Muffins

2 cups barley flour
½ cup oat flour (or oat bran)
½ cup whole-wheat flour
2 tsp. all-phosphate baking powder
½ tsp. salt
1 Tbsp. safflower oil (optional)
2½ cups milk

Mix dry ingredients. Stir in (oil and) milk—add more milk if necessary. Spoon into greased muffin tins and bake at 425 degrees about 25 minutes or until light brown.

Makes 16 muffins at 133 calories each
Protein 13%; carbohydrate 77%; fat 10%.

Sat. fat	.19 gm.	Cholesterol	.78 mg.
Mono. fat	.13 gm.	Fiber	.94 gm.
Poly. fat	.64 gm.	Sodium	136 mg.

Variations: Oat flour and/or whole wheat flour can be omitted for an all-barley muffin. Reduce milk to about 2 cups.

Appetizers, Salads, and Vegetables

Mideastern Yogurt

This is often served in Lebanese or other Mideastern restaurants along with hummus and tabouleh as appetizers. You can use pita bread to scoop it with. We often order two or three of the appetizers as dinner when we find a Mideastern restaurant.

1 small cucumber, chopped finely
2–3 cloves garlic, minced
2 cups plain nonfat yogurt

Mix ingredients together thoroughly.

Makes 4 half-cup servings at 76 calories
   each
Protein 36%; carbohydrate 60%; fat 4%

Sat. fat	.15 gm.	Cholesterol	2 mg.
Mono. fat	.06 gm.	Fiber	1.1 gm.
Poly. fat	.05 gm.	Sodium	89.3 mg.

Cabbage Salad or Low-Oil Coleslaw

This is our almost daily winter salad. Cabbage is very nutritious. In fact, daily doses of salted cabbage (sauerkraut) kept early sailors from getting scurvy. If you buy preshredded cabbage and carrots, the salad takes only minutes to make.

1 lb. cabbage, shredded (can be purchased shredded in most supermarkets)
1 or 2 carrots, shredded or sliced
2 tsp. olive oil
Dash of salt (⅛ tsp.)
¼–½ tsp. garlic powder (optional)
Pepper to taste
1–2 tsp. lemon juice or vinegar (optional)

Mix all ingredients and toss well to distribute oil (or put in a covered container and shake). Flavor improves after an hour or so and it keeps well for several days, especially if you do not add lemon juice or vinegar or add only as you serve.

Makes 9 1-cup servings at 28.73 calories each			
Protein 10%; carbohydrate 58%; fat 32%			
Note: Fat content by percentage appears to be high because the overall calories are so low.			
Sat. fat	1.6 gm.	Cholesterol	0 mg.
Mono. fat	.74 gm.	Fiber	1.5 gm.
Poly. fat	.14 gm.	Sodium	69.2 mg.

Variations:
1. Add Italian seasonings, bean sprouts, or if you're not trying to lose weight, 1 Tbsp. of toasted pumpkin or sunflower seeds.
2. Add diced green peppers.
3. Add a diced tomato when you're ready to serve.

Zucchini Salad

3–4 zucchini, sliced
1 large tomato, diced
1 green pepper, diced
1 small sweet onion or red onion, chopped or in rings
1 tsp. salt
Pepper to taste

Mix all ingredients. Refrigerate for several hours. The salt draws moisture from the squash and the salad creates its own "sauce" or salad dressing. Keeps several days. (Add basil or Italian seasonings if desired.)

Makes 8 servings at 15 calories each		
Protein 19%; carbohydrate 73%; fat 8%		
Sat. fat .03 gm.	Cholesterol	0 mg.
Mono. fat .02 gm.	Fiber	1.2 gm.
Poly. fat .1 gm.	Sodium	247.1 mg.

Steamed Vegetables

You can, of course, simmer vegetables in a little water or cook them in the microwave, but nothing preserves the flavor (and nutrients) like steaming. And nothing could be easier.

If you don't have one, get a collapsible stainless steel steamer basket (about $4.00). Many woks come with a steamer-plate on which you can steam vegetables with fish.

Put water in bottom of a pot to just below the steamer. Put fresh or frozen vegetables in the steamer, cover tightly, and bring water to a boil, steaming vegetables until just tender. (If you mix vegetables, add quicker-cooking ones last.)

Enhance, if desired, with any of the following:

1. Season with defatted butter buds (available in supermarket or in bulk in natural food stores). One type can be sprinkled on, another mixed with warm water for a sauce.
2. Sprinkle vegetables like broccoli with lemon juice or add lemon juice to defatted butter and water mixture.
3. Sprinkle with Mrs. Dash, pepper, or a little salt.

4. Add dill weed to carrots or green beans, nutmeg to spinach.
5. Drizzle vegetables with a little olive oil, then add a little basil and garlic powder.

Main Dishes

Broiled Fish

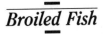

There is nothing easier to cook than broiled fish. I only include the recipe in case you're new in the kitchen. (Even Bryant could do this.)

16 oz. fish fillets (catfish, perch, haddock, snapper, salmon, etc.)
Seasonings to taste (see variations below)

Arrange fish on a flat pan that has been lightly greased. Cook under the broiler about 6–8 inches below heat for about 6–8 minutes. Turn and cook for another 2–5 minutes, depending on thickness of fillets. Fish is done when it flakes easily with a fork. Try not to overcook. Serve with slices of fresh lemon and steamed vegetables for a quick and easy meal.

Makes 3 servings of sole or flounder at 176 calories each
Protein 88%; carbohydrate 0%; fat 12%

Sat. fat	.55 gm.	Cholesterol	102.4 mg.
Mono. fat	.47 gm.	Fiber	0 gm.
Poly. fat	.62 gm.	Sodium	158.3 mg.

3 servings of haddock at 169 calories each
Protein 92%; carbohydrate 0%; fat 8%

Sat. fat	.25 gm.	Cholesterol	112.1 mg.
Mono. fat	.23 gm.	Fiber	0 gm.
Poly. fat	.47 gm.	Sodium	131.6 mg.

3 servings of salmon at 279 calories each
Protein 62%; carbohydrate 0%; fat 38%

Sat. fat	2.1 gm.	Cholesterol	74.7 mg.
Mono. fat	4.0 gm.	Fiber	0 gm.
Poly. fat	3.3 gm.	Sodium	88.9 mg.

Variations:
1. Sprinkle fish with garlic powder, Mrs. Dash, and lemon juice before broiling.
2. Marinate fish in the refrigerator for an hour or more, in 3–4 Tbsp. lemon juice and seasonings like rosemary, sage, and thyme—or in lemon juice, garlic, and basil—or in lemon and dill or tarragon.

Easy Creole Fish

16 oz. firm white fish
1 16-oz. can tomatoes, diced or whole
1 green pepper cut in rings or chopped
1 large onion, sliced
1 bay leaf
1 tsp. thyme
3 Tbsp. basic roux (see recipe, page 256)

Combine all ingredients except fish in a deep pan. (Break up whole tomatoes.) Simmer until pepper and onions are tender. Add fish and gently simmer 10 minutes or until fish flakes easily with a fork. Add pepper or Tabasco and a little salt to taste. Serve over brown rice if desired.

---

4 servings at 218 calories each (no rice)
Protein 53%; carbohydrate 23%; fat 24%.

Sat. fat	.94 gm.	Cholesterol	94.7 mg.
Mono. fat	2.9 gm.	Fiber	2.4 gm.
Poly. fat	1.1 gm.	Sodium	336.7 mg.

4 servings at 450 calories (with 1 cup brown rice).

Sat. fat	.94 gm.	Cholesterol	94.7 mg.
Mono. fat	2.96 gm.	Fiber	88 gm.
Poly. fat	1.1 gm.	Sodium	336.7 mg.

Easy Fish Loaf

We like this better with mackerel than with salmon, but if you prefer a non-fishy taste, you might like the salmon.

1 small onion, chopped or minced
2 Tbsp. green pepper, chopped
3 Tbsp. dried parsley (or minced fresh)
2 Tbsp. lemon juice
2 slices whole-wheat bread, torn in small pieces
1 tsp. olive oil
½ cup skim milk
2 tsp. basil
¼ tsp. garlic
¼ tsp. salt
1 16-oz. can of mackerel or pink salmon, drained

Combine ingredients and mix well. Cook in greased loaf pan for 25 minutes at 425 degrees, or until lightly brown.

Preparation time: 8–10 minutes.

Makes 4 servings at 227 calories each
Protein 45%; carbohydrate 20%; fat 35%.

Sat. fat	2 gm.	Cholesterol	.6 mg.
Mono. fat	2.9 gm.	Fiber	1.99 gm.
Poly. fat	2.4 gm.	Sodium	858.8 mg.

Variations:
1. Substitute 1 cup oats or oat bran for whole-wheat bread crumbs. (Makes 4 servings at 275.5 calories.)
2. Add (or substitute) 2 Tbsp. celery or chopped olives.

Quick Salmon Salad

1 16-oz. can pink salmon (or mackerel)
¾ cup skim cottage cheese
1–2 stalks celery, diced
1 small onion, minced or diced

Mix all ingredients. Add a little garlic powder, pepper, or Mrs. Dash, if desired.

> Makes 3 servings at 264 calories each
> Protein 58%; carbohydrate 7%; fat 35%.
>
> | Sat. fat | 2.7 gm. | Cholesterol | 2.5 mg. |
> | Mono. fat | 2.9 gm. | Fiber | .71 gm. |
> | Poly. fat | 3.2 gm. | Sodium | 1091 mg. |

Variations:
1. Substitute nonfat yogurt for cottage cheese.
2. Add: 1 can water chestnuts, sliced
       1 Tbsp. capers
       1 tsp. dill, fresh or dried
3. or 1 small apple, diced, and ¼ cup raisins, celery
4. or 1 cup pineapple chunks (in natural juices or fresh) with celery or water chestnuts
5. or 8 olives, chopped

Use your imagination and whatever you have on hand: a few garbanzo beans, sunflower seeds, etc.

Sautéed Chicken with Vegetables

2 boned and skinless chicken breasts (16 oz.)
½ tsp. olive oil
¼ tsp. garlic powder or 2–3 garlic cloves, minced
1 10-oz. pkg. frozen whole baby carrots
1 10-oz. pkg. frozen whole petite green beans or sugar-snap peas
Salt and pepper to taste

Slice chicken breasts into small strips. Heat oil and garlic powder in skillet over medium high heat. Sauté chicken strips about 8–10 minutes or until done. Remove chicken strips from frying pan to a warm plate. (If you cook in a wok, you can move chicken to one side while you cook carrots and beans.) Place one package of whole baby carrots and sauté in leftover drippings from chicken. Add a little water and simmer, loosening cooked drippings from bottom of pan. Add one package of petite green beans and heat for another 4–5 minutes. Return chicken to skillet. Heat through and serve with brown rice, if desired.

Total preparation and cooking time for chicken and vegetables: 20 minutes.

Makes 4 servings at 223 calories each
  (without rice)
Protein 68%; carbohydrate 13%; fat 19%.

Sat. fat	1.2 gm.	Cholesterol	96.3 mg.
Mono. fat	1.8 gm.	Fiber	3 gm.
Poly. fat	.92 gm.	Sodium	107.1 mg.

Variations:
1. Add 1 diced onion and 1–2 cups sliced cabbage to carrots and beans.
2. Substitute any of your favorite vegetable combinations.

Chicken or Turkey Gumbo

Of all the things I cook, this is probably Bryant's favorite. And he hates okra. In Mobile, Alabama, where I grew up, and all along the Gulf Coast, every cook's gumbo is different. Some use more roux or lighter roux or more crab. Some cook it so long that you can't tell what you're eating. My mother's gumbo looks like mud, and it tastes wonderful. Many gumbos include sausage or ham. This is a lipo-fitness version.

2 stalks celery, chopped
1 or 2 onions, chopped
1 or 2 green peppers, chopped
3 Tbsp. basic roux (see recipe, page 256)
1 lb. (more or less) leftover cooked chicken or turkey in pieces
  (white meat)

1 10-oz. pkg. chopped okra
1 16-oz. can tomatoes
2–3 cups fat-skimmed chicken stock (optional)
Parsley
1 bay leaf
Tabasco sauce

Sauté onions, celery, and peppers in olive oil. Add roux and other ingredients. Add water to make about 4 quarts. Simmer for several hours or until okra has fallen apart. Season to taste with a little Tabasco and salt. Serve over a mound of brown rice in a large soup bowl.

> Makes 16 1-cup servings (without rice) at 85
>   calories each
> Protein 51%; carbohydrate 26%; fat 24%.
>
> Sat. fat   .44 gm.   Cholesterol 24.06 mg.
> Mono. fat   1 gm.   Fiber   1.0 gm.
> Poly. fat   .36 gm.   Sodium   73.2 mg.

Variations: If available, add a couple of crab bodies to initial ingredients. They will impart a wonderful flavor. You can also add shrimp, oysters, or crabmeat either initially or about ½ hour before serving. Many Southern cooks put everything in to begin with and cook it all day—so that all the flavors blend together. But if you want to see your shrimp or oysters, put them in later. You can also sprinkle a tsp. of filé (ground sassafras leaves) over each bowl before serving. Traditionally, either filé or okra is used as a thickening agent.

Lemon/Basil Chicken

4–5 Tbsp. lemon juice
½ tsp. powdered garlic (or 2–3 cloves, minced)
2 tsp. basil
½ tsp. salt
1 Tbsp. olive oil
2 chicken breasts, boneless and skinless (16 oz.)
Non-aerosol cooking spray

Mix all ingredients except chicken, crushing basil and garlic with back of spoon. Add chicken breasts cut either into 4 pieces or thinly sliced. Marinate at least an hour in the refrigerator. Remove chicken from marinade and sauté in a pan sprayed with cooking spray. Pour marinade over chicken and simmer a few minutes. (Add 1 Tbsp. arrowroot or cornstarch to thicken if desired.)

Makes 4 servings if served with whole-wheat pasta or 2 8-oz. servings served with steamed vegetables. (Spinach or broccoli and carrots are good.)

Makes 4 servings at 208 calories each
  (without pasta or vegetables)
Protein 71%; carbohydrate 6%; fat 23%

Sat. fat	1.3 gm.	Cholesterol	96.3 mg.
Mono. fat	3.0 gm.	Fiber	.2 gm.
Poly. fat	0.9 gm.	Sodium	83.5 mg.

Variations:
1. Add ½ cup sliced mushrooms and/or several green onions after sautéing chicken. If you're short on time you can make it without marinating the chicken.
2. You can use chicken breasts with bones. Remove the skin before marinating and cooking.

Basic Pasta Dishes

Cook 8–16 oz. whole-wheat spaghetti or other whole-wheat pasta until tender. Drain.
   Eat with:

1. Basic meatless spaghetti sauce, homemade or commercial, to which you might add microwaved or sautéed mushrooms, green peppers, onions.
2. Eat with cottage cheese if desired. (See Easy Pasta and Cottage Cheese recipe.)
3. Warm 1 Tbsp. olive oil and a little minced or powdered garlic in a large bowl. Add 8 oz. cooked pasta and toss. Add a few pine or other nuts, black olives, and 1 Tbsp. Parmesan cheese. Toss and serve. Or add 2 chopped anchovies, 1 Tbsp. capers. Or fresh mushrooms, chopped tomatoes and basil. (Create your own variations.)

Serving of 1 cup spaghetti with 1 cup sauce,
   mushrooms, and green peppers: 470
   calories
Protein 10%; carbohydrate 66%; fat 24%

Sat. fat	1.7 gm.	Cholesterol	0 mg.
Mono. fat	6.1 gm.	Fiber	1.4 gm.
Poly. fat	3.3 gm.	Sodium	1.238 mg.

Serving of 1 cup spaghetti with ½ cup sauce,
   mushrooms, and green peppers: 334
   calories
Protein 11%; carbohydrate 70%; fat 19%

Sat. fat	.87 gm.	Cholesterol	0 mg.
Mono. fat	3.1 gm.	Fiber	1.39 gm.
Poly. fat	1.687 gm.	Sodium	620 mg.

Easy Pasta and Cottage Cheese

8 oz. whole-wheat or whole-wheat spinach pasta
1 cup cottage cheese
Dash of garlic powder
Pinch of basil
2 cups meatless spaghetti sauce

Cook and drain noodles. Mix garlic and basil with cottage cheese. To
serve, put cottage cheese over noodles and cover with spaghetti sauce.
Heat in microwave (or heat sauce on stove before adding).

Makes 2 servings at 368 calories each
Protein 17%; carbohydrate 65%; fat 18%

Sat. fat	1.2 gm.	Cholesterol	2.5 mg.
Mono. fat	3.2 gm.	Fiber	1.8 gm.
Poly. fat	1.6 gm.	Sodium	848 mg.

Italian Stuffed Shells

1 24-oz. container low-fat cottage cheese, well drained
1 10-oz. pkg. frozen spinach, thawed and well drained
½ cup grated Parmesan cheese
¼ tsp. garlic
1 tsp. basil
1 egg
1 10-oz. pkg. Italian shells or manicotti
2 cups meatless spaghetti sauce

Combine first six ingredients. Cook and drain pasta according to package directions. Stuff with cheese mixture. Pour a little spaghetti sauce in bottom of baking dish and spread. Arrange stuffed pasta on dish. Cover with remaining sauce. Bake in 375-degree oven about 25 minutes.

Makes 4 servings (6 shells per person) at 326 calories each		
Protein 20%; carbohydrate 68%; fat 12%		
Sat. fat 1.2 gm.	Cholesterol	21.5 mg.
Mono. fat 1.3 gm.	Fiber	1.6 gm.
Poly. fat .5 gm.	Sodium	403.2 mg.

Fettucine

1½ cups low-fat cottage cheese
1 cup skim milk
½ tsp. garlic powder
1 tsp. basil
1 tsp. olive oil (optional)
¼ tsp. salt (optional)
1 8-oz. can minced clams, drained (optional)
16 oz. whole-wheat spaghetti or other pasta
Parmesan cheese

Put first five ingredients in a blender and process for a few seconds to make sauce. Add clams to sauce, but do not process in blender. Cook pasta. While pasta cooks, heat sauce gently—do not boil.

Put pasta on plates. Spoon cheese mixture over it. Sprinkle 1 tsp. Parmesan cheese over each dish if desired.

Total working and cooking time: 15–20 minutes.

Makes 6 servings at 337 calories each		
(without Parmesan)		
Protein 25%; carbohydrate 67%; fat 9%		
Sat. fat	.63 gm.	Cholesterol	26.9 mg.
Mono. fat	.74 gm.	Fiber	1.2 gm.
Poly. fat	.08 gm.	Sodium	356.6 mg.

Variations:
1. Omit clams and add 1 can drained salmon and 1 Tbsp. capers and do not heat. Toss with cooled noodles and serve.
2. Add a 16-oz. can of water-packed artichokes, drained, to sauce (omit clams). Serve hot or cold.

Basic Roux

I grew up on the Gulf Coast where a roux is the basis for wonderful gumbos, other seafood dishes and beans. Traditionally roux is made from half fat and half flour, but the low-oil version works fine. A good roux ranges in color from a golden dark brown to very dark brown but not burned.

1 Tbsp. olive oil
3 Tbsp. whole-wheat flour

Mix oil and flour in a heavy pan. Over medium-low heat, stir until roux is dark brown. Gradually add a little water until roux is dispersed and add to beans, gumbos, or other dishes.

Creole Red Beans and Rice

In New Orleans, my friend Cynthia's mother always had a pot of red beans on the back of the stove. It was traditionally Monday night dinner and a side dish the rest of the week. Waldo, Cynthia's father, said you couldn't have dinner without red beans.

Basic Roux (see page 256)
4 cups dried red kidney beans (about 32 oz.)
1 tsp. garlic powder (or 2–3 cloves, minced)
1 green pepper, chopped
1 large onion, chopped
2 stalks celery, chopped
1 tsp. of each or some of the following: basil, thyme, oregano, marjoram
1 bay leaf
2 Tbsp. parsley
1 tsp. salt
½ tsp. crushed red peppers or pepper or Tabasco sauce to taste

Wash beans and soak overnight in 4 quarts water. Boil, then simmer until beans are tender (about 3 hours). Add water, if necessary (to replace water lost to evaporation), to make 2½ –3 quarts. Add roux.

Sauté green pepper, onions, and celery, in a pan sprayed with cooking spray, add them and seasonings to beans. Simmer for about an hour. (Mash a few beans against the side of the pot to make gravy thicker.) Serve over brown rice. Makes about 3 quarts.

Makes 12 1-cup servings of beans at 230
  calories each
Protein 24%; carbohydrate 69%; fat 7%

Sat. fat	.27 gm.	Cholesterol	0 mg.
Mono. fat	.89 gm.	Fiber	7.18 gm.
Poly. fat	.49 gm.	Sodium	176.9 mg.

1 cup beans and ½ cup brown rice = 345
  calories
Protein 19%; carbohydrate 75%; fat 6%

Sat. fat	.27 gm.	Cholesterol	0 mg.
Mono. fat	.89 gm.	Fiber	10.4 gm.
Poly. fat	.49 gm.	Sodium	176.9 mg.

Mexican Bean Cornbread

Toppings:

2 16-oz. cans navy beans, drained and rinsed
10-oz. can chopped tomatoes with green chilies
1 onion, diced
1 green pepper diced (optional)
2 cups cottage cheese
½ tsp. garlic

Cornbread:

1½ cup stone-ground corn meal
½ tsp. baking soda
1 tsp. all-phosphate baking powder
½ tsp. salt (optional)
1 cup milk

Heat oven to 500 degrees.

Mix first four topping ingredients and simmer for a few minutes while you mix cornbread. Mix cottage cheese and garlic together.

Cornbread: Mix dry ingredients, add milk. Pour into a deep 9″ pie pan greased with margarine or cooking spray. Put in oven for 8 minutes. Remove and spread with a layer of cottage cheese and then a layer of the bean/chili mixture. Bake for another 10–12 minutes. Slice into 8 wedges.

Working time: about 20–25 minutes.

Makes 8 servings at 262 calories each			
Protein 29%; carbohydrate 64%; fat 7%			
Sat. fat	.53 gm.	Cholesterol	3.438 mg.
Mono. fat	.22 gm.	Fiber	6.2 gm.
Poly. fat	.1 gm.	Sodium	547.2 mg.

Stir-Fry Zucchini

Garlic powder or several garlic cloves
2 tsp. olive oil
2–3 zucchini, sliced
1 green pepper, sliced
1 onion, cut in large pieces
1 tomato, cut in large pieces

Heat garlic in oil. Add zucchini, pepper, and onion and stir-fry a few minutes. Add tomatoes and continue to cook until zucchini is just tender. Add a little water if necessary. Add a dash of salt. Serve with brown rice. (Add ground sesame seeds to rice to get complete protein, or eat with garbanzo, navy, or other beans.)

Makes 6 servings; each serving with 1 cup brown rice: 266 calories Protein 9%; carbohydrate 81%; fat 10%			
Sat. fat	.25 gm.	Cholesterol	0 mg.
Mono. fat	1.1 gm.	Fiber	8 gm.
Poly. fat	.22 gm.	Sodium	3.6 mg.

Lentil Salad

1 lb. lentils, washed
3 small onions, chopped
½ tsp. garlic powder (optional)
1 Tbsp. olive oil
2 tsp. lemon juice or vinegar
1 tsp. basil
1 stalk celery, chopped
1 green pepper, chopped
Fresh or diced parsley

Combine lentils and onions (and garlic, if desired) and cover with water. Cook until just tender (about 20 minutes). Use these, drained and cooled, as a basis for a summer salad.

For salad, combine 3 cups of the cooked lentil mixture with the
remaining ingredients.

Makes 3 servings at 263 calories each			
Protein 24%; carbohydrate 61%; fat 15%			
Sat. fat	.66 gm.	Cholesterol	0 mg.
Mono. fat	3.32 gm.	Fiber	10.68 gm.
Poly. fat	.45 gm.	Sodium	76.63 mg.

Mushroom and Rice and Bean Salad

2 cups fresh mushrooms, sliced
4 green onions, sliced
1 cup cooked brown rice
1 cup cooked beans (navy, garbanzo, lentils, etc.)
¾ cup cottage cheese (or nonfat yogurt)
¼ tsp. garlic or 1–2 garlic cloves, minced (optional)
Mrs. Dash or pepper, to taste

Mix ingredients.

Makes 5 1-cup servings at 122 calories each			
Protein 29%; carbohydrate 66%; fat 5%			
Sat. fat	.24 gm.	Cholesterol	1.5 mg.
Mono. fat	.10 gm.	Fiber	3.82 gm.
Poly. fat	.06 gm.	Sodium	150.7 mg.

Variations:
1. If you don't have cooked rice on hand, make with 2 cups of drained
   and rinsed canned beans and eat whole-wheat bread to complement
   protein in beans.
2. Make with all brown rice. Add ground sesame seeds to complement
   the protein in the rice.

Cottage Cheese Salad

1 cucumber, chopped
1 tomato, chopped
1 cup low-fat cottage cheese
1 cup alfalfa sprouts
¼ tsp. garlic powder
¼ tsp. pepper

Mix all ingredients together thoroughly.

Makes 4 1-cup servings at 60 calories each		
Protein 52%; carbohydrate 36%; fat 12%.		
Sat. fat	.41 gm.	Cholesterol	2.5 mg.
Mono. fat	.18 gm.	Fiber	1.76 gm.
Poly. fat	.12 gm.	Sodium	234.1 mg.

Variations: Add or substitute any fresh salad vegetable: carrots, zucchini, celery, green pepper, etc.

Banana/Pineapple Cheese Salad

2 bananas, peeled and cut up
1 16-oz. can pineapple chunks, in natural juices
2 cups low-fat cottage cheese
1–2 Tbsp. sunflower seeds (optional)

Mix ingredients. Sprinkle a few sunflower or pumpkin seeds on top.

Makes 4 servings at 200 calories each (when made with 2 Tbsp. sunflower seeds)		
Protein 31%; carbohydrate 53%; fat 16%		
Sat. fat	1.1 gm.	Cholesterol	5 mg.
Mono. fat	.79 gm.	Fiber	2.33 gm.
Poly. fat	1.6 gm.	Sodium	461.1 mg.

Makes 4 servings at 174 calories each
  (without sunflower seeds)
Protein 33%; carbohydrate 59%; fat 8%

Sat. fat	.84 gm.	Cholesterol	5 mg.
Mono. fat	.37 gm.	Fiber	2.33 gm.
Poly. fat	.12 gm.	Sodium	461 mg.

Artichoke Hearts and Cheese Salad

1 16-oz. can artichoke hearts (packed in water), drained
2 cups low-fat cottage cheese
2 grapefruit or 1 16-oz. can pineapple chunks (in natural juices)

Mix artichoke hearts and cottage cheese. Peel grapefruit and divide into segments or drain pineapple and serve on top of and around cottage cheese mixture.

Makes 4 servings at 172 calories each
Protein 38%; carbohydrate 55%; fat 7%

Sat. fat	.78 gm.	Cholesterol	5 mg.
Mono. fat	.35 gm.	Fiber	4.78 gm.
Poly. fat	.15 gm.	Sodium	535.2 mg.

Lentil Soup

1–2 large onions, diced
½ –1 cup celery
3–4 cloves of garlic or 1 tsp. garlic powder
2 tsp. olive oil
2 cups brown lentils, washed and drained
1 cup sliced carrots
1 tsp. basil
1 16-oz. can of tomatoes
4 quarts water
½ cup dried parsley or 1 cup fresh parsley
Salt and pepper to taste

Sauté onions and celery with garlic powder in olive oil. Add washed and drained lentils, carrots, basil, canned tomatoes, and water to fill a 4-quart pot. Bring to a boil; reduce heat and simmer for approximately 30 –40 minutes. Add parsley. Season to taste with pepper and a little salt.

Working time: 15 minutes.

Makes 16 servings at 101 calories
Protein 28%; carbohydrate 64%; fat 8%

Sat. fat	.13 gm.	Cholesterol	0 mg.
Mono. fat	.47 gm.	Fiber	.96 gm.
Poly. fat	.20 gm.	Sodium	62.36 mg.

Variations:
1. Add ½ to 1 cup of any of the following: corn, green beans, chopped cabbage, or other vegetable.
2. If you're low on vegetables, add ¼ cup pearled barley or brown rice.
3. If you like the flavor of curry, omit basil and add 2 tsp. (or more) of curry powder and 2 Tbsp. lemon juice and a little cumin or Tabasco.
4. Add 1 Tbsp. Bako yeast a few minutes before serving. It is a nutritional yeast that imparts a smoked bacon flavor. (Available in natural food stores.)

Quick Bean Soup with Green Chilies

2 16-oz. cans Great Northern or navy beans
½ tsp. garlic powder (or 2–3 minced cloves)
1 tsp. olive oil
1 onion, chopped
2–3 Tbsp. chopped, canned green chilies

Sauté onion and garlic in oil for just a few minutes. Put one can of beans in the blender for a few seconds. Add it to onions and garlic. Add the other can of beans, 2–3 Tbsp. of chopped green chilies (or more to taste). Add a little water to make soup desired thickness and heat. *Note*: To reduce salt, rinse canned beans or use dry cooked beans.

Good served with Corn/Wheat Muffins or corn tortillas and slaw.

Makes 2 large servings at 574 calories each
Protein 24%; carbohydrate 58%; fat 7%.

Sat. fat	.35 gm.	Cholesterol	0 mg.
Mono. fat	1.7 gm.	Fiber	23.2 gm.
Poly. fat	.26 gm.	Sodium	92.4 mg.

Easy Salmon Soup

This is one of our favorite winter soups. It is quick and easy and nutritious.
It's also good with roux added (see basic Roux recipe, page 256).

1 large onion, chopped
1 green pepper, chopped
1–2 stalks celery, chopped (optional)
½ tsp. garlic powder or 2–3 garlic cloves, minced
1 Tbsp. olive oil
1 16-oz. can tomatoes
1 tsp. basil (optional)
1 16-oz. can chicken broth with fat skimmed off (optional)
1 16-oz. can salmon (or mackerel)
Parsley

Sauté onion, pepper, celery, and garlic in olive oil. Add tomatoes, basil,
chicken broth. (Substitute water if you do not have broth.) Simmer for
15 minutes. Add salmon, a handful of parsley, and heat well. Add a
little water if thinner soup is desired.

Preparation time: about 10 minutes.

Total working and cooking time: about 30 minutes.

Makes 4 servings at 210 calories each
Protein 46%; carbohydrate 18%; fat 36%

Sat. fat	2.0 gm.	Cholesterol	0 mg.
Mono. fat	3.0 gm.	Fiber	2.0 gm.
Poly. fat	2.6 gm.	Sodium	832.7 mg.

Easy Red Bean Soup

1 onion, chopped
3 stalks celery, chopped
2 tsp. olive oil
1 Tbsp. whole-wheat flour
2 cans red beans, drained (or 2 cups cooked red, pinto, Anasazi
    or other beans)
2 bay leaves
1 tsp. paprika
½ tsp. garlic powder (optional)
1 tsp. lemon juice
Tabasco sauce

Sauté onions and celery in oil. Add flour, and stir until smooth. Add
beans, bay leaves, paprika, garlic powder (if desired), enough water to
bring to desired consistency, and lemon juice. Simmer for about 20
minutes. Put in blender for a few seconds; season with a dash of
Tabasco sauce. (As canned beans are already salted, you'll probably not
need additional salt.)

Working time: 10–15 minutes.

Makes 4 1-cup servings at 213 calories each		
Protein 20%; carbohydrate 64%; fat 16%		
Sat. fat	.36 gm.	Cholesterol	0 mg.
Mono. fat	1.7 gm.	Fiber	7.3 gm.
Poly. fat	.29 gm.	Sodium	443.9 mg.

Vegetable and Bean Soup

Just about any vegetables can be used to make a soup. I find, however,
that a turnip adds a distinctive flavor that we miss when it's not there. In
the winter, I usually put a pot of soup on the woodstove on Saturday
morning and let it simmer all day.

2 onions
2 stalks celery
1 Tbsp. olive oil
1 large turnip, diced
2–3 carrots
2–3 cups sliced cabbage
1 can tomatoes
1/3 cup brown rice or pearled barley (optional)
1/2–1 cup green beans
1 1/2 tsp. garlic powder
1 tsp. basil
1 tsp. salt
1 can beans (garbanzo, pinto, Great Northern), drained
  (optional)
1 1/2 Tbsp. dried parsley (or 1/4 cup fresh, chopped)

Sauté onions and celery in oil. Put all ingredients, except beans, in a 4-quart pot. Add water to cover. Bring to a boil and then simmer for an hour or two. Just before serving add beans and a handful of dried or fresh parsley.

> Makes 4 quarts—16 1-cup servings at 60
>   calories each
> Protein 12%; carbohydrate 69%; fat 19%
>
> | Sat. fat | .15 gm. | Cholesterol | 0 mg. |
> | Mono. fat | .64 gm. | Fiber | 2.4 gm. |
> | Poly. fat | .14 gm. | Sodium | 263.5 mg. |

Variations:
1. Add ½ cup dried Anasazi beans initially and omit canned beans.
2. For a more nutritious variation, add ½ cup of arami, kelp, or other seaweed for added vitamins and trace minerals.

Desserts

Rice Pudding

5 cups cooked brown rice
2 eggs or 1 egg and 2 egg whites
2 cups skim milk
1 Tbsp. honey or brown sugar
2 tsp. cinnamon
1 cup raisins

Place cooked rice in a 9 × 9 or 9 × 12 pan. Beat eggs with fork; add skim milk, honey, and cinnamon. Sprinkle raisins over rice. Pour milk mixture over rice.

Bake at 325 degrees for 45 minutes to 1 hour or until center is firm and top is lightly browned.

Makes 10 half-cup servings at 171.4 calories
  each (with whole eggs)
Protein 12%; carbohydrate 79%; fat 9%

Sat. fat	.44 gm.	Cholesterol	55.8 mg.
Mono. fat	.48 gm.	Fiber	3.7 gm.
Poly. fat	.17 gm.	Sodium	41.8 mg.

Variations: Substitute cooked pearled barley for brown rice for a chewy texture.

Quick Apple Dessert

This is especially easy to make if you have an apple corer/slicer, a round gadget with a center hole and spokes radiating out. Place it over an apple, press down, and you have 8 perfect slices, immediately cored.

4 Golden Delicious (or other) apples, cored and sliced
1 Tbsp. raisins
1 Tbsp. walnuts

1 Tbsp. lemon juice
Cinnamon to taste

Place apples and raisins and walnuts in a glass dish. Sprinkle with lemon juice and cinnamon. Cover and microwave on high about 5 minutes. Or bake in a conventional oven at 375 degrees about 15 minutes or until apples are tender.

Makes 4 servings with raisins and walnuts
    at 98 calories each
Protein 3%; carbohydrate 87%; fat 10%

Sat. fat	.1 gm.	Cholesterol	0 mg.
Mono. fat	.2 gm.	Fiber	3.5 gm.
Poly. fat	.6 gm.	Sodium	1.6 mg.

Blackberry Crisp

1 cup oats
½ cup whole-wheat flour
1 Tbsp. corn oil margarine, melted
2 Tbsp. brown sugar
4 Tbsp. skim milk
3 cups berries

Mix all ingredients except berries. Put berries in a baking dish and crumble mixture over them. Bake at 425 degrees about 15 minutes or until lightly browned.

Good as is, or serve with skim milk or low-fat yogurt.

Makes 4 servings at 240 calories each
Protein 10%; carbohydrate 72%; fat 17%

Sat. fat	.8 gm.	Cholesterol	.3 mg.
Mono. fat	2.1 gm.	Fiber	9.8 gm.
Poly. fat	1.1 gm.	Sodium	44.3 mg.

Variations: Substitute apples and cinnamon, peaches, or other fruits and berries.

Not-So-Short Cakes with Strawberries

2 cups whole-wheat pastry flour
2 tsp. baking powder
½ tsp. salt (optional)
2 Tbsp. safflower oil
2 Tbsp. honey
⅔ cup skim milk

Mix dry ingredients. Mix oil, honey and milk and add. Stir until a soft batter is formed. Drop onto cookie sheet or knead a few times, then pat out flat and cut out rounds with a biscuit cutter or inverted glass. Bake at 450 degrees for 12 minutes or until lightly browned. Serve with strawberries and skim milk if desired.

Makes 10 cakes at 124 calories each
   (shortcakes only—no strawberries)
Protein 12%; carbohydrate 66%; fat 22%

Sat. fat	.4 gm.	Cholesterol	.3 mg.
Mono. fat	.3 gm.	Fiber	3.1 gm.
Poly. fat	2.1 gm.	Sodium	143.8 mg.

Pineapple Upside-Down Cake

2 Tbsp. liquid or melted corn-oil margarine
2 Tbsp. brown sugar
1 16-oz. can pineapple slices or chunks (juice packed), drained
1 Tbsp. safflower oil
½ cup honey
1 whole egg and 2 egg whites
½ cup plus 1 Tbsp. skim milk
1 tsp. all-phosphate baking powder
¼ tsp. salt
1 cup whole-wheat pastry flour

In an 8″ or 9″ baking pan, heat margarine and coat pan. Add brown sugar and arrange pineapple evenly over sugar and margarine mixture.

Beat oil, honey, eggs, and milk together. Mix baking powder, salt, and whole-wheat flour and add to liquids. Beat to smooth consistency. Pour the batter over the pineapple mixture. Bake at 325 degrees for 35–40 minutes or until wooden toothpick inserted in center comes out clean. Allow to cool for about 10 minutes and invert on serving plate.

Makes 9 servings at 184 calories each		
Protein 8%; carbohydrate 68%; fat 23%		
Sat. fat .8 gm.	Cholesterol	30.7 mg.
Mono. fat 1.9 gm.	Fiber	2.2 gm.
Poly. fat 1.8 gm.	Sodium	160.9 mg.

Index